S. T. CLARK'S®

great
MELALEUCA
fact book

Published By:

Gaughan Fisch, Inc.
1666 White Bear Avenue, Box 291
St. Paul, Minnesota 55106

Seventeenth Printing – May, 1997

The personality behind the author is that of a "retired" freelance writer, business writer, poet and journalist who has spent the majority of his working life in and around the writing and printing businesses.

BOOKS BY S.T. CLARK®

Published by Gaughan Fisch, Inc.:
    S.T. Clark's® Great Melaleuca Fact Book

Published by Compton Park Companies, Inc.
    S.T. Clark's® Diabetes & Melaleuca Alternifolia Oil
    S.T. Clark's® Health To Wealth
    S.T. Clark's® How Safe Is Your Home

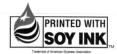

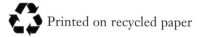 Printed on recycled paper

Printed in the United States of America   ISBN: 0-9639521-0-2

CONTENTS

TESTIMONIALS

"My 15 year-old daughter complained of leg cramps for over a year before I joined Melaleuca. I'd hear her call for me during the night and I'd run to her room and massage the leg having the cramp. I never failed to tell her what my mother told me when I had similar leg cramps - "It's growing pains; you're a tall person and steadily growing taller. Leg cramps are to be expected when one is growing as fast as you are." Well, now she takes one Mel-Vita® and one Mela-Cal® daily; within less than two months after starting these, she never experienced any more leg cramps. Now, I believe the cramps were caused by a vitamin deficiency. Please understand that I am a mother who tries to provide a minimum of two well-balanced meals daily for my children. Typically, however, I'm not sure about their lunches."

- J.V., Florida

"To clean my make-up and cosmetic brushes, I just add a few drops of Tough 'N Tender™ in a sinkful of warm water. It works every time! I also use 1/2 teaspoonful Tough 'N Tender™ in a 16-ounce spray bottle filled with water as an insect repellent on my plants; this same combination works well as a cleaner on our silk plants, too. Also, I want to respond to your reference (in cleaning veggies) about assuming that the water from your kitchen faucet is safe. Well, let me tell you: in most areas of this country, it isn't. But that's another story and as you say, another book."

- M.T., Minnesota

"Here's my Melaleuca story: I was opening my desk drawer and pulled it out too far; it dropped on my foot right below my big toe. There was a break in the skin and my foot started to turn black and blue; I could easily see where the break was! I grabbed my bottle of T36-C7® and rubbed a generous amount on my foot; I followed this by rubbing in liquid Pain-A-Trate®, too. The pain went away nearly immediately and the swelling went down. The black and blue also disappeared. Several hours later, I did my regular 2-1/2 mile walk with no trouble. When I later looked at my foot, I couldn't find where the skin was broken! My foot was still slightly puffy, so I rubbed some more Pain-A-Trate® on. Melaleuca oil is just amazing; I had thought that I had broken my foot - the pain was that intense. And after just a couple of applications, I was good as new! You know, without Melaleuca oil (and a great product containing the oil), I would have been off my feet for a week!"

- M.M., Florida

FOREWORD

THE WORDS THAT FOLLOW are the result of a lifelong commitment to reporting both the common and the uncommon.

I have learned that writing in its purest form is a solitary pursuit where one stares at an empty page waiting for words to materialize. On rare occasions they appear as nearly finished copy; most times, however, they come as only draft beginnings. There is no glamour in this part of the writing experience; there is only mystery and self-doubt. While the physical act of writing is solitary, any writer's work comes from a collaboration where all knowledge acquired and all experiences generated become the references and influences that combine with new thoughts to form the words and opinions expressed.

Throughout this book I have tried to keep explanations and terminology in a language easy for both of us to understand. I am neither physician nor scientist. Even though I lack medical credentials, I am well-experienced in research, reporting facts, and the necessary fundamentals associated with writing for publication. This fact-filled book is not based on emotional hype, half-baked theories, or an excess of self-serving mumble-jumble no one but the author can understand. The name of this book best describes its contents: S.T. Clark's® Great Melaleuca Fact Book.

This book, first introduced in mid-November, 1993, has been revised for the 3rd time and is now in its 15th printing. Over the months, I have resisted adding sections describing "other" Melaleuca products. After all, this is a book on the oil and products containing the oil; not an advertisement for any particular company's products. Yet after taking super-antioxidants consistently for the last few months, I have begun to understand how important they can be to my own general health. Since super-antioxidants offer dramatic hope for those suffering from heart and circulatory conditions, arthritis and memory loss, and non-infectious diseases like diabetes, I now feel compelled to add a chapter devoted to this most amazing non-oil product. You'll also note other changes and small additions throughout this book; some changes and (hopefully) improvements continue in nearly every edition.

This book is dedicated to all of those who helped in the preparation and editing, and to those who gave me rest and companionship throughout my life's journey. Each owns part of my humble thanks and lasting gratitude.   - S. T. Clark®

TESTIMONIAL

"I'm prone to developing yeast infections, and in the fall of 1992, I had a real bad case. The doctor gave me several different types of medications to try. However before any worked, the infection had spread throughout my entire groin area and up on my stomach. It produced real deep wounds or sores, and none of the prescribed medicine was effective in healing me. Soon I was nearly bedridden and receiving in-home nursing care.

At Christmas we were invited to a relative's home in southeastern Minnesota. By this time, I was more ambulatory and using heavy bandages to cover my open sores. My cousin, a Melaleuca representative, brought along some product samples for me to try. My, how we all fell in love with Melaleuca's lotions! He told me to use Melaleuca's Antibacterial Liquid Soap™ when washing my sores and to then apply T40-C5™ Oil of Melaleuca and Mela-Gel™ to the open wounds.

My doctor ordered daily visits by a registered nurse. When she came, I told her I wanted to use the Melaleuca products. She said, 'Sure, I use Melaleuca products, too.' So twice a day, my sores were washed with Antibacterial Liquid Soap™ and air dried with a cool hair dryer. In only a few days, the open sores started healing and coming together.

By the way, my doctor gave his approval for the use of Melaleuca products. He had recently told the nurse that unless these wounds healed, I would need surgery and a large part of my stomach would be removed because the sores were so deep. Meanwhile, the sores kept getting better, so we started washing with a few drops of both Sol-U-Mel™ and Natural Spa & Bath Oil™ added to water. We also continued to apply T40-C5™ and Mela-Gel™.

Complete healing was achieved in about two months; now I have beautiful baby-like skin where once I had such an outbreak of open and infected sores. I also apply Body Satin™ Lotion after my bath each day - my skin is so nice from using this lotion! And I continue to routinely use Antibacterial Liquid Soap™, even though I no longer have any infection. I still sometimes get yeast infections and find that Nature's Cleanse™ alleviates them right away.

I'm sorry this letter is so long, but I just wanted to tell everyone how sold I am on Melaleuca's products. My registered nurse will also verify how effective Melaleuca oil has been for me. Together, we can clearly proclaim that Melaleuca alternifolia oil was completely successful in helping heal me. Thank you Melaleuca, and thank you for allowing me this space to tell my story in S.T. Clark's™ Great Melaleuca Fact Book."

-Mrs. E.H., Minnesota

2

INTRODUCTION

SEVERAL YEARS AGO while visiting friends in southeastern Minnesota, I was introduced to an oil they called their "miracle in a bottle." They told me the oil eased the stiffness in arthritic joints, relieved migraine headaches and healed cuts and rashes. They also showed me how the oil could immediately relieve the sharp pain from a bee sting (gained while touring their strawberry patch). After applying a few drops of this oil, the pain vanished and the bite area did not become red or swollen. The bottle of oil was labeled T36-C7™ Oil of Melaleuca. Before that afternoon, I had never heard of this product. However, the words "Melaleuca alternifolia oil" were soon woven into my everyday language, becoming central topics of ordinary conversation.

While my friends knew only some basic information about Melaleuca alternifolia oil, I needed to know more. As someone who always looks for a story, I was determined to delve into "all things Melaleuca." I was anxious to find out if this miracle oil could alleviate a wide variety of ailments that affect the world's population. If Melaleuca alternifolia oil ended pain and misery with the ease I had seen, I wondered what other benefits were common to the oil, and what else it could heal.

The reason I have written this book is to give voice to "what else the oil could heal." Many of the "else's" uncovered are nothing short of incredible. This book was written then, to bring together under one cover as much practical data on Melaleuca alternifolia oil as could reasonably be assembled.

If you have ever attempted to find information on the subject of Melaleuca from your local library, you probably can understand my initial frustrations in working to complete this manuscript. Even the prestigious University of Minnesota Medical School's library offered only limited data. Yet time and persistence paid off and a variety of reference materials and reports were assembled. Combined with the personal testimonials from independent product users, they form this book.

We also have good news to report to the estimated 16,000,000 diabetics living in the United States and Canada - because with Melaleuca, there really is good news! When you finish reading this book, I'm confident you'll realize that while every possible use hasn't been mentioned, the included information could well represent **the most complete collection of Melaleuca alternifolia oil information available anywhere under one cover.**

If you know of a product use that is not mentioned here, or if you have found something that works better than what I have suggested, why not write me a note? If your testimonial is used in a future edition, a complimentary copy of that edition will be sent to you. This is my personal guarantee.

Melaleuca alternifolia oil is effective on such a variety of conditions because the oil is penetrating, soothing, aromatic and non-caustic. It also is a natural fungicide, a natural solvent and a natural antiseptic.

I hope you will share what you learn in these pages with those you know and those you love. Personally, I have found that a person has everything to gain and nothing to lose when sharing their knowledge with others.

Tell everyone you know about Melaleuca alternifolia oil. Loan this book to friends and family, or buy them their own copy. Note the money-saving multiple copy discounts on the inside back cover. S.T. Clark's® Great Melaleuca Fact Book is an excellent gift for birthdays and anniversaries, graduations, special events, and at the holidays a copy makes an ideal "stocking stuffer".

The method you use to acquire this book, whether you borrow it, buy it, or even find it, is not nearly as important as having a personal copy to read and use as a reference. When you finish reading this book, I'm confident that you will join hundreds of thousands of others who now proclaim that "Melaleuca alternifolia oil is truly the miracle oil in a small bottle".

WORDS OF CAUTION

CAUTION #1: Any product use or course of treatment suggested in these pages should not be considered a substitute for obtaining appropriate medical care when and where needed. If you have a serious medical problem or illness always consult your physician or primary care-giver well before beginning a new program or before altering any prescribed or existing course of treatment. Proper choices regarding your health and well-being will enhance your life. Remember, doing nothing is also making a choice.

CAUTION #2: I have included a wide variety of suggested product uses under the "Chore List" and "Farm Facts" sections. The reader is reminded that "suggested uses" are based upon my personal experiences and the experiences of others I know. As in most circumstances, individual results will vary. I have often found that using less of a product, rather than more, will sometimes give better results. Other factors that may cause a difference in results can include the water's temperature, quality (city-supplied, spring or well), degree of hardness or softness and proper measurement and mixture of product.

CAUTION #3: Products containing Melaleuca alternifolia oil generally work well on almost everyone, however, there are exceptions. Melaleuca alternifolia oil provides tremendous healing benefits unlike any other products. But, it will not always provide the same benefits for everyone.

People who suffer from contact dermatitis should not use the pure oil. It has been noted that even if results indicate this condition is initially helped by applications of the **pure oil**, in time the condition will deteriorate and worsen. I would caution anyone with any type of dermatitis to proceed very slowly in their treatment. However, I have seen several people with very serious cases of contact dermatitis find relief with Problem Skin Lotion™. This appears to have a very positive healing effect when consistently used.

Those allergic to fragrances may also experience problems, as some Melaleuca products do contain fragrances. Many do not, however, so read the labels carefully and use accordingly.

Knowing yourself and being aware of possible or potential problems before they happen is your safest assurance. It is always important to consider that Melaleuca alternifolia oil-based products, as with any products, are not universal cure-alls that work the same for everyone. Understanding what your own body can effectively use and tolerate certainly beats carrying a rabbit's foot, particularly for the rabbit.

CAUTION #4: Insist on knowing exactly what you are buying and using. Also insist on knowing the product's source and manufacturer. While Australia has uniform testing standards for Melaleuca alternifolia oil, the United States (at this writing) does not. The requirement to use only the alternifolia tree when producing Melaleuca oil is now regarded as essential by the Australian Tea Tree Industry Association. These products are distributed by other companies, or are available in the general retail marketplace. While products may be labeled as containing 100% Tea Tree Oil, or even 100% Melaleuca Oil - and may contain oil from Melaleuca or Tea trees, their oil may still not be 100% pure Melaleuca alternifolia oil. With hundreds of different Melaleuca trees, only the Melaleuca alternifolia tree produces the healing and beneficial effects found in pure Melaleuca alternifolia oil.

Always insist on buying Melaleuca alternifolia products from reputable sources. These products are distributed by other companies, or are available in the general retail marketplace. While products may be labeled as containing 100% Tea Tree Oil, or even 100% Melaleuca Oil - and may contain oil from Melaleuca or Tea trees, their oil may still not be 100% pure Melaleuca *alternifolia* oil.

NAME CALLING

"MELALEUCA ALTERNIFOLIA" is the botanical name for a shrub-like tree belonging to the Myrtle family native to New South Wales, Australia. The tree grows naturally wild in the lowland areas around the Clarence and Richmond River systems. Now, domesticated, it is grown on huge plantations located in the same general area.

Traditionally, medicine has relied on plants for its source of drugs. The public's demand for natural medicinal products, like oil produced from the Melaleuca alternifolia tree, has increased in recent years. Melaleuca oil reportedly contains dozens of different compounds that work in synergy. Some are so unique they are found nowhere else in nature.

Some people use the term "tea tree oil" when referring to Melaleuca alternifolia oil; others refer to it as "ti oil." In this book, I use the terms "Melaleuca oil" or "Melaleuca alternifolia oil" interchangeably. Sometimes when I think you know what I am referring to, I will just use the word "oil." But most times, I will call the tree by its full botanical name: "Melaleuca alternifolia", and refer to the oil as "Melaleuca alternifolia oil."

The name you choose to call this oil is not really that important. What is important is that you remember that Melaleuca alternifolia oil is a natural substance. All the research and documentation I've thus far studied, indicates that this oil is of a higher quality than any other naturally occurring substance.

TESTIMONIALS

"I'm a diabetic and often suffer from severe foot and leg sores that always seem difficult, if not impossible, to fully heal. In the past my doctor has prescribed both strong prescription pills and ointments in an attempt to help heal and alleviate some of my worse sores. Other than taking my regular insulin injections three times daily, I don't like taking drugs. And, I've also had problems in not being able to tolerate many of the strong ointments she has prescribed.

Until a friend gave me a copy of your book, I had assumed there was no practical solution that could really help me. So first, I want to tell you how grateful I am that you published S.T. Clark's™ Great Melaleuca Fact Book!

Third, your book mentions there are some [15,000,000 of us (diabetics) in the U.S. and Canada]. In my limited circle of contacts, I probably know at least 40 to 50 other diabetics who could be helped by Melaleuca oil. Oh yes, I skipped the second item I wanted to tell you - I wanted to save it for last. I have enrolled as a Melaleuca preferred customer and already have received my 3rd shipment of products. I plan to order every week! Best of all, my foot and leg sores are healing. I am so grateful to you and your book - and of course, to Melaleuca. Thank you so much for my renewed health!"

-L.B., **Texas**

"I have discovered another effective treatment for hemorrhoids. After a warm bath, I apply Mela-Gel™ to the entire area. It provides a nice lubricating and cooling effect. Plus, it helps reduce the painful inflammation. My job requires me to sit at a desk and often deliver work to other offices; sometimes I am in intense pain when required to be on my feet or to stand for extended periods. However, I've found that applying Mela-Gel™ frequently throughout the day helps ease the pain while it heals the acute soreness.

As a word of caution, since we have several containers of Mela-Gel™ around our house, I've learned to label mine with an "H". This way, everyone knows the "H" container is used for treating a special problem area. You won't believe the complications and chaos it caused in my home when I forgot to properly label my personal Mela-Gel™ container!"

-B.R., **Florida**

The History of
Melaleuca Alternifolia Oil

BEFORE SUMMARIZING THE HISTORY of Melaleuca alternifolia oil, it is probably best to briefly give some background information about Australia, the land where the oil is believed to have originated. Australia, the largest island in the world, is often referred to in our admittedly romanticized view as "the land down under." However, modern Australia had a most unromantic beginning. It was developed primarily because the British had a crime problem. Following the American Revolution, the Crown could no longer send undesirables and rebels to America. The English searched for, and found, an even more remote and out-of-the-way land, known since ancient Greece and Rome as *terra australis incognita*, to become their newest holding area for convicts and unwanted political prisoners.

Eons ago, Stone Age people lived in caves and tents constructed from tree branches and leaves. These Aborigines are believed to have reached Australia after sailing from parts of the Asian mainland. Some people now suggest that all Australians were originally boat people who came to the shores of the continent from virtually every part of the globe.

Captain James Cook's explorations determined that Australia was separated by sea from New Guinea. However, in claiming possession of the eastern lands for his King, he did not know if the west coast and the east coast were joined, or if they were two separate islands.

After Cook's return to England, the British started adding to Australia's population by sending their dissidents. These new arrivals came primarily to New South Wales. Ireland contributed its rebels, Scotland gave its free spirits, and thieves were sent from England. All were given one-way passage.

Australia was not the lush tropical land many in the northern hemisphere believed. In his book, *The Australians*, author Ross Terrill notes that even Charles Darwin commented, "...The gum trees were miserable-looking and presented the appearance of being actually dead...[Their] rivers are without water, trees give no shade, flowers are without perfume, and birds such as the emu can't fly." He also is quoted, "Although Captain Cook had reported that Botany Bay was fertile and abundant, this was an explorer's excess of enthusiasm, and for two decades the struggle for food was acute."

Australia is somewhat less rough and tumble today. It is still known for a hearty outback lifestyle, independent thinking, and peculiar (to those of us in the northern half of the globe) climactic contrasts. The southern regions are closer to the Antarctica and relatively cool. The northern areas have tropical climates and are home to rare vegetation like the Melaleuca alternifolia tree. It grows wild in the swamps and in the low-lying, flood-prone areas.

Captain Cook reportedly noted that Aborigines brewed a spicy tea from the aromatic and sticky leaves they picked from a shrub-like tree. Some leaves were used to treat internal problems and some were used to crush and cover wounds and injuries. Captain Cook is credited with discovering, for the modern world, this tree that one day would be botanically named the *Melaleuca alternifolia*. He named it the *Tea Tree*.

Historical reports and writings make scant mention of uses for Melaleuca alternifolia leaves or oil during the one hundred fifty-plus years following Captain Cook's expeditions in the 1770's. Dr. A.R. Penfold, an Australian government chemist, rediscovered the oil in the 1920's. He is credited with being the first modern-day chemist to study Melaleuca alternifolia oil. Dr. Penfold found that the oil, when used as an antiseptic bactericide, was 10 to 12 times stronger than carbolic acid, the antiseptic then considered standard. Dr. Penfold reported, "[Melaleuca alternifolia oil] is particularly recommended as a non-poisonous, non-irritant antiseptic and disinfectant of unusual strength [having] valuable antiseptic properties. [The] spicy flavoring should prove useful in dentifrices and mouthwashes."

In 1930, Dr. E.M. Humphrey, an Australian scientist, reported in *A New Australian Germicide*, "[Results] were excellent....Infections which had resisted treatments of various kinds for months were cured in less than a week. Twenty drops in a tumbler of warm water, used as a gargle, quickly cleared up a sore throat in the early stages. [The oil's] action on typhoid bacilli has been found to be more than 60 times as rapid as other so called disinfectant soaps. It is an excellent deodorant and immediately clears away any foul smell from wounds or abscesses. It [is] an excellent prophylactic for infective conditions which gain entrance to the body."

The *Medical Journal of Australia* reported in 1930 that Melaleuca alternifolia oil was effective in curing septic wounds. The most striking feature of the oil was that it dissolved pus and left infected wound surfaces clean. The germicidal action was very effective. There was no apparent damage to the tissue from the oil. This report also suggested that localized tissue infections would favorably respond to the oil and the benefits would include wound sterilization, decreased complications and increased rates of healing.

An Australian medical journal reported in 1936 that oil from the Melaleuca alternifolia tree successfully treated diabetic gangrene and prevented subsequent limb amputation.

In the years since 1936, independent research documented the uses of Melaleuca alternifolia oil and verified its unique ability to penetrate deeply into tissues, end infection and leave surfaces healthy. Since the oil is virtually non-toxic, it was found to be valuable in surgical and dental procedures, and in treating conditions of the mouth and throat. Because of these qualities, it was widely used and recommended by the Australian medical community. They found that the oil could penetrate and help sterilize infected wounds, heal and prevent septic, and eliminate infection and pus. Pharmacies routinely dispensed Melaleuca alternifolia oil to treat insect bites, infected wounds, skin cuts and abrasions.

With an increasing number of conditions responding to Melaleuca oil applications, the public's demand exceeded producers' supplies. Production often proved impossible because weather conditions in some years were too severe to allow harvesting. Since Melaleuca alternifolia trees grew wild in low-lying areas, heavy rainfall and high water levels meant low yields, inadequate supplies and inconsistent quality.

When so-called wonder drugs, including penicillin, were introduced in the mid-1940's, the world's medical community became fascinated with drugs that could be manufactured in cost-effective environments. Most medical practices gravitated to these new remedies for treating even minor conditions. New treatment options were aggressively promoted by drug companies, as physicians recommended over-the-counter and prescription medicines. This led to a revolution in medical care where even minor complaints would be treated with drugs and more frequent visits to the doctor. Soon, natural products were considered to be *old fashioned relics* and new products were thought to hold the *promise of the future*. Profit-driven pharmaceutical companies marketed new drugs aggressively, promoting their synthetics as the universal answer to nearly every medical problem.

The cycle of times in the 1940's continued to spin through good times and bad until it reached a full turn. As in many turnings, people often look back to see if they can find what it was they left behind. During this long period beginning in the 1940's and stretching into the early years of the 1980's, the use of Melaleuca alternifolia oil declined significantly. As demand for the oil declined, pharmacies no longer stocked it. Prices increased, therefore, only those willing to pay the increased price purchased the oil.

Despite the higher prices, some continued to use Melaleuca alternifolia oil. Limited research discovered new treatments and new application successes. In the years following Dr. Penfold's studies, dozens of published reports recognized the intrinsic value of the oil in treating various conditions. These reports appeared in internationally recognized medical journals, magazines and periodicals. *The United States Dispensatory* reported that Melaleuca alternifolia oil was actively germicidal.

Approximately 30 years ago, Dr. Eduardo F. Pena studied the oil's effectiveness in eradicating vaginitis and candida albicans. His research found the oil to be a penetrating germicide and fungicide that effectively dissolved pus and debris. In his study group of 130 test patients, all reported success using Melaleuca alternifolia oil.

From the 1970's into the 1980's, several Australian concerns developed Melaleuca alternifolia tree plantations. Growing trees on huge plantations enabled producers to ease climactic harvesting restrictions. Domesticated trees grown in controlled environments meant the quality of the oil produced would be consistent, prices would be stable, and sufficient quantities would be available to meet anticipated world-wide demands.

In the 1980's, Melaleuca alternifolia oil was again *rediscovered* - this time by Americans who brought the oil to the United States. Brothers Roger and Allen Ball, along with Frank Vandersloot, founded Melaleuca, Inc., a consumer-direct marketing company that produces a line of products containing Melaleuca alternifolia oil. The company reportedly will use oil only from trees never exposed to pesticides or herbicides.

A February, 1991 letter in *The Lancet* stated that, "[Melaleuca alternifolia oil] has antibacterial properties that might make it a valuable alternative remedy for the treatment of acne... I would like to report a patient in whom [the] oil seemed to cure anaerobic vaginosis... I am unaware of any previous reports in which [Melaleuca alternifolia oil] has been used for this condition, but this anecdotal case indicates that this herbal remedy should be assessed..."

A 1992 article, "Systemic contact dermatitis from tea tree oil" by Anton C. DeGroot and J. Willem Weyland of The Netherlands, in *Contact Dermatitis* reported, "A patient [who had] long-standing atopic dermatitis, who was sensitized to tea tree oil from its application to atopic dermatitis as an "alternative" medicament; after initial improvement, the patient suspected that the dermatitis was becoming worse from the medicament. He was then advised to ingest the oil mixed with honey. This resulted in obvious exacerbation of the dermatitis."

(Note: This above report seems to be opposite to almost every suggested use that advocates Melaleuca alternifolia oil as a topical application only. This information is included, then, for informational purposes only, to inform the reader that studies of a variety of potential applications continue in some of the world's leading medical research facilities.)

Melaleuca alternifolia oil is now used and recommended by a growing number of health-care professionals including dentists, physicians, veterinarians, chiropractors and therapists. Worldwide, Melaleuca oil is used by tens of thousands of ordinary citizens and professionals to treat an increasingly large variety of conditions and ailments. The preceding pages described only a few of the hundreds of scientific studies performed on the Melaleuca alternifolia tree's leaves and oil. Study conclusions demonstrate time and again that leaves from the Melaleuca alternifolia tree produce an extremely beneficial oil that can well be referred to as one of Nature's most powerful antiseptics.

As our future continues to be written, the future uses for Melaleuca alternifolia oil continue to be discovered. Think of the impact the oil is having with dairy farmers and with those concerned with animal husbandry. Certainly the previously mentioned studies must not have anticipated most of these new uses. Yet with any product brought to the marketplace, those who individually comprise that marketplace determine the usefulness and true success of the product introduced. As a growing number of consumers discover the oil, new applications will also continue to be discovered. It is a fact that Melaleuca alternifolia oil has produced amazingly successful results in study after study. It is these results, and the differing numbers of practical uses for Melaleuca alternifolia oil, that are the reasons for the writing and publishing of *S.T. Clark's® Great Melaleuca Fact Book.*

TESTIMONIALS

I just wanted to tell you how pleased we are about [S.T. Clark's™] Great Melaleuca Fact Book. You've captured exactly the information we need to become more effective in telling the Melaleuca product story. Speaking of stories, I just love the way S.T. Clark weaves his stories around Melaleuca's facts. It makes me eager to read this book's facts and turn the pages to see what's been written, there. What a wonderful book this is! Now, for the first time, I am able to read and really understand the value of Melaleuca and why their products will indeed enhance my life. I hope my "thank-you's" don't appear too trite. They come from my heart. So, thank you!
                                                                    -T.R., **Colorado**

"My family has avoided coming down with both the colds and serious flu that almost everyone around here seems to have caught this past year. Whenever one of us first has a tickle warning - the one in the back of their throat - or a sore throat that seems to be coming on, we reach for the Melaleuca products and go to work. I've found that gargling with Breath-Away™ mouthwash is an excellent start; for best results, I let a little of it "trickle" down my throat as I gargle. I have another treatment that really works too: I put 2 to 3 inches of water in a heavy sauce pan and bring it to a rolling boil, then I remove the pan from the heat and put on a hot pad at the table. Next, I add 1 to 2 capfuls Sol-U-Mel™ and then breathe the steam in through my nose and turn my head sideways to exhale through my mouth. For me, it works best if I continue this until the pan has stopped steaming. This has really worked to relieve my head stuffiness, too. I generally repeat the procedure every 2 to 3 hours.

By following this simple procedure and recipe, I've found that all my stuffiness and possible flu and potential cold symptoms stay as symptoms only, and soon disappear. I don't know what's in Melaleuca that makes it work so well on so many different things, but whatever it is, I've come to just accept it as another one of our Lord's blessings. I'm old enough to know that I don't have to understand how something works in order to realize that it just plain works. But, you don't have to take my word for this. Someday, if you're developing symptoms of a cold or flu, why not try this yourself and see if it can work for you, too?"   *-B.P.,* **North Carolina**

"This is the best Melaleuca book I've seen, and the only one I'll now recommend. Not only have you given information on hundreds of personal care and household uses, but you've also brought us an abundance of farm and diabetic care data, too. Certainly, this IS the finest Melaleuca information book available."   *-R.B.,* **Minnesota**

14

HARVESTING AND PRODUCTION FACTS

NOW THAT YOU HAVE READ something about the discovery, research and history of Melaleuca alternifolia oil, it is probably also important to learn how one country's trees have grown into such a modern-day miracle for so many people throughout the world.

The Melaleuca alternifolia tree is a hearty, paper-barked shrub-like tree that generally grows to heights under 20 feet. Leaves are harvested twice annually in a process that leaves the trees undamaged and available for new growth and future harvesting. Producers report that regular cuttings of leaves and branches stimulate, rather than retard, the natural growth of the trees.

Melaleuca alternifolia oil is obtained in a distillation process where steam passed through leaves ruptures the tiny oil cells. This creates a vapor that, when condensed, forms a liquid that passes through tubes surrounded by cold water. The liquid then drains into holding tanks where the lighter-than-water oil floats on the surface where it is skimmed off and collected.

Because of harvesting difficulties, producers were forced to develop alternative growing procedures. Select trees were transplanted and large plantations were established that would guarantee a consistent quality of oil and adequate supplies to meet market demands. The only task then, was to recreate market demand.

Plantation owners funded research programs to determine new uses for the oil. They realized that if their markets could be expanded, demand would increase as other uses were developed. Research indicated that the oil produced beneficial results when used in veterinary medicine, as an additive for cleaning products, lawn and tree fungi treatments, and in alleviating a diverse number of medical and dental conditions.

Melaleuca alternifolia trees are now grown in several parts of the world outside Australia, including Spain, Portugal and some areas of the United States. Some people have suggested that one day Melaleuca alternifolia may become California's most important farming revenue source and the state's largest export.

AN ANALYSIS OF
MELALEUCA ALTERNIFOLIA OIL

THE QUALITY OF MELALEUCA ALTERNIFOLIA OIL is determined by high concentrations of terpinen-4-ol (up to 60%) and low concentrations of cineole (less than 10%). Cineole is a skin irritant and the major property of eucalyptus oil. Terpinen-4-ol is considered the primary therapeutic agent. Its interaction with the other compounds is believed to be significant in the ability of the oil to deliver the healing action so consistently demonstrated.

Studies have determined that Melaleuca alternifolia oil contains some properties not found anywhere else in nature. Additional research indicates the oil is 4 to 5 times stronger than ordinary household cleaners and disinfectants. Generally, it does not sting when it is applied to minor cuts and abrasions.

Melaleuca, Inc. offers two pure oil products. T36-C7™ contains 36% terpinen and 7% cineole; T40-C5™ contains 40% terpinen and 5% cineole.

WORDS OF RECOMMENDATION

TO ASSURE THAT THE Melaleuca alternifolia oil products you purchase are of the highest quality, it is most important to use a reputable source. There are several choices and alternative sources to consider when contemplating the purchase of any products containing Melaleuca alternifolia oil.

When I began my research into the oil, I studied several companies and researched as many products as was reasonably possible. By doing this, I was then able to determine which one - in my personal opinion - was the best company and which company offered the best product line. I tried to be openly objective to my task. As a writer, I was interested in discarding the "fluff" and "getting to the meat". In order to endorse any particular product line, I needed to be absolutely sure that my endorsement would be based on the facts as I would learn them *and not on a "story" that someone may have wanted an inquiring mind to believe*. In order to recommend a particular manufacturer, it was critical that I be more than satisfied with both the company selected and their product line. On a more personal level, it was essential that my family, friends and others who might one day read my words, would also accept my recommendations. Giving an opinion to others, known and unknown to me, involves accepting risk and at the least, some potential for embarrassment. However, with everything I learned about the company I selected and now recommend, any risk is nearly non-existent. There also is, I believe, little opportunity for my choice to cause anyone any embarrassment.

Melaleuca, Inc. is the only company that I can personally recommend. I sincerely believe that my family, friends and everyone else will benefit from their "dealings" with this company. I have been a Melaleuca customer for almost two years. I can assure anyone that this company is unique. Personally, I have found Melaleuca, Inc. to be uncompromised by greed and unswerving in loyalty to their customers. Proof of this is evidenced in the quality of their offered products, dedication of staff, and a refund and return policy that far exceeds that of any other manufacturer.

Melaleuca's marketing method also impressed me. Generally, their 80-some products are not sold in retail stores. The company calls itself, "America's only consumer-direct marketing company". When I enrolled, I wanted to buy my products wholesale, so I became an insured (now termed a "preferred") customer. I simply call Melaleuca's 800 number to order whatever products I want. My order is quickly shipped directly to me via UPS. It's so simple that anyone can do it. And there's never a hassle and rarely a mistake. However when one occurs, the company's response is truly amazing.

Let me tell you about the only problem I have ever experienced with a Melaleuca order. Several years ago around Christmas, I ordered a bottle of Melaleuca's finest perfume. It was packaged in a cedar box. When my ordered arrived, the box had a small "nick". I called Melaleuca's customer service number and expected the traditional run-around I had experienced in dealing with other companies. Imagine my surprise when the customer service representative apologized and offered to replace the perfume. When I asked how I should send the first one back, she told me to keep it for my trouble. Wow!

When I first started my independent study of Melaleuca oil and products containing the oil (as produced and/or distributed by Melaleuca, Inc.), there seemed to be only "clusters" of its customers scattered throughout America. Well, times have indeed changed! Now there seemingly are hundreds of thousands of Melaleuca customers located in every section and corner of the United States and in most of Canada as well.

Throughout these areas you'll find folks who mirror you and I - people just like most of us who introduce their neighbors, family and friends to the shopping-from-home method of Melaleuca's consumer direct marketing program. Many of these home shoppers have discovered how easy it really is to obtain all of their household and personal care products **cost-free each month** by simply introducing ten friends who will also commit to using Melaleuca's at-home shopping for the purchase of their products, too.

I don't know anyone who shouldn't become a Melaleuca customer; I don't know anyone who shouldn't use and advocate the use of Melaleuca's products. My advice therefore is that if you are not already a customer, talk with another customer in your area. If someone has given you this book to read, talk to them. They will show you how you can become a preferred customer, buy Melaleuca products wholesale and convert your home and life from harmful store-bought stuff to Melaleuca's safe and effective concentrated (low cost per use) products. I have found that Melaleuca people are almost everywhere, in every community. I know one would be delighted to talk with you.

If you're a shy person, someone unable to find someone, ask someone you trust, someone around your area. Many Melaleuca people are shy too; they're just like us, people who try to stay nearly invisible to the naked eye, ones largely unable to make contact with others. But, persevere, be brave and ask around.

However, if you've gone through all the motions, have asserted yourself, researched your community and still can't find anyone on your own, you can contact us. We'll then try to put you in touch with someone close to you. Reading S.T. Clark's® Great Melaleuca Fact Book is a good beginning step. The next step is telling someone you want to learn more about Melaleuca's marketing opportunities. *So, whether you're a shy person or someone who's outgoing, a bubbly sales leader looking for something to enhance your life or someone so shy you're as thin as a rail because you can't talk in the grocery store - the decision to make that first call is really is up to you! If you were sitting across the table from me right now, I'd just tell you to, "Go for it!!" The only thing you have to lose is your future good health. . .*

NOTE: While this book specifically recommends products manufactured by Melaleuca, Inc., *this book has NOT been authorized or approved by that company. This book is NOT a Melaleuca (Inc.) sponsored publication.*

TESTIMONIALS

"I am a registered nurse here in Rochester. Our 9-year old daughter's leukemia is in remission now, but she still suffers from the result of an infection she had during her chemotherapy which resulted in the loss of her sphincter muscle. Doctors recently did surgery to repair this problem. Upon her return home from the hospital, we cleaned the entire bathroom with Sol-U-Guard™ to prevent infection. We had to irrigate her wound each time she stooled (about 12 times daily), and we used the tub for this. I would clean the tub with Sol-U-Guard™ after each time; it kills germs and leaves the room smelling clean. At one of her recent weekly check-ups, her doctor said it looked like she had a yeast infection near her wound created by the surgery. He wrote a prescription for a cream to kill the infection. I then showed him my Mela-Gel™ (he had not heard of it) and asked if he thought it could help since it was antibacterial and anti-fungal. He told me to use it or his prescription for the cream. I applied Mela-Gel™ regularly for a week until her next appointment. At that visit, the doctor was "amazed" at her progress and asked me what I'd used. I told him more about Melaleuca and about my Mela-Gel™ and Anti-Bacterial Liquid Soap™ which we also use for her bath."   **-S.J., Minnesota**

"This is "our recipe" for a Melaleuca-style first aid mixture we keep in our medicine chest and first-aid kits. Making it up ahead of time means it will be available for wound cleansing when it's needed. In a 16 ounce spray bottle, we combine 2 ounces Sol-U-Mel™ and 2 to 3 drops T36-C7™. Rather than depending on the quality of regular tap water, we prefer using distilled water. This spray works really well on almost any wound or injury.

Living out here in the country, it seems that someone is always needing some sort of treatment for some type of problem or injury. When something occurs, we do this: (1) In a small bowl, use 2 full squirts of Anti-Bacterial Liquid Soap™ and (2) fill with distilled water; (3) then use a sterile dressing pad to gently wash the wound before (4) flushing with more distilled water (to clean out any foreign or decayed matter); (5) next, spray the special solution (from the preceding paragraph) before (6) gently patting the area dry with a sterile cloth.

We use ordinary cotton swabs to apply Triple Antibiotic Ointment™ on and around a wound's general area. When healing starts, we apply Mela-Gel™ at least 3 to 4 times daily. Our best results come when we stay with this treatment schedule and even continue to treat the area for a week or so after it has fully healed. So, we use Body Satin Lotion™, or Problem Skin Lotion™ or Hand Creme™ on the (former) injury, having found that the steady use of these products really helps keep the skin supple and soft."   **-S.K., Colorado**

CONDITIONS RESPONDING
TO MELALEUCA ALTERNIFOLIA OIL

REPORTS TELLING OF PROFESSIONAL PRACTICES that use Melaleuca alternifolia oil are steadily increasing. This writer knows of dentists, veterinarians, and clinical staffs who privately, and now more publicly, advocate the use of products containing Melaleuca alternifolia oil.

With the new emphasis on the oil, it is interesting to note that scientists have reportedly been unable to synthetically duplicate Melaleuca alternifolia oil. They have discovered that even when they were successful in synthesizing most of the active compounds, the substance they produced was less potent and more toxic than the oil in its natural form.

Products containing Melaleuca alternifolia oil are accepted today and used increasingly by those choosing natural options as opposed to synthetically produced chemicals.

Hundreds of thousands of people from all walks of life, having all sorts of differing histories and experiences, now routinely use the pure oil and products containing Melaleuca alternifolia oil, for alleviating and often healing these conditions:

Chapped Hands	Abrasions
Bed Sores	Boils & Carbuncles
Acne	Halitosis
Oral Thrush	Itchy & Flaky Skin
Allergic Rashes	Cuts & Scrapes
Dandruff	Dental Decay
Cradle Cap	Congestion
Insect Bites	Coral Cuts
Sore Throat	Hemorrhoids
Bleeding Gums	Canker Sores
Burns	Warts
Rough Skin	Stinging Nettles

Vaginitis
Scabies
Poison Oak
Arthritis
Sports Injuries
Migraine Headaches
Gum Disease
Ear Aches
Sinusitis
Gingivitis
Head Lice
Muscle Aches
Chicken Pox
Pruritis
Rashes
Shingles
Sinus Congestion

Corns
Poison Ivy
Poison Sumac
Sunburn
Sprains
Jock Itch
Ear Infection
Athlete's Foot
Cold Sores
Chapped Lips
Ingrown Toe Nails
Paronychia
Psoriasis
Diabetic Foot Ulcers
Red Eye
Ringworm

As you read through the following pages and find a condition I have missed, please let me know. **Or,** if your suggested treatment differs from mine, I would like to know that, too. If your suggestion is the first like it that I receive and is used in a subsequent edition, you will receive a complimentary copy of the first book in which it appears.

THE FACTS: INFECTION, HUMAN SKIN AND THE IMMUNE SYSTEM

I REALIZED DURING MY RESEARCH into *all-things-Melaleuca*, that the variety of medical conditions alleviated by using the oil should be investigated. This broad-titled chapter is written to discuss healing results that are both amazing and profound.

With the public's attention focused on diseases represented by various charitable groups, perhaps the greatest medical problem facing the world is unrepresented by any general charity. This wide-spread killer is infection. While deaths from diabetes, cancer and heart disease steadily increase each year, deaths attributed to infection now lead all other causes. Despite the progress of the scientific community in developing new drugs to treat symptoms, science seems to be at a loss when it comes to developing effective treatments to eradicate infectious diseases.

During the last 60 years, antiseptics used in surgery have significantly reduced morbidity rates. Less than 100 years ago, if surgery was required, the patient had about a 50-50 chance of survival.

I come from a family line of frugal Norwegians on one side and equally frugal Scots on the other. Both families shared one thing in common - a passion for living that often stretched life well into nine decades and sometimes a little more - all of it lived alive (there IS a difference between living alive and mere living). They were self-medicated, self-sufficient, generally sober and God-fearing. However, my grandfathers on both sides died in their early thirties, following non-antiseptic surgery for conditions that today would be considered minor and even routine.

With basic antiseptic programs that included thorough hand washing and maintaining antiseptic environments, survival rates increased as dramatically as the overall progress and development of modern medicine. Today, we're witness to a growing number of clinical staffs, hospitals, nursing homes, physicians, dental practices, chiropractors, therapists and veterinarian offices that routinely use and advocate the use of Anti-Bacterial Liquid Soap™. This liquid soap is antibacterial and contains Melaleuca alternifolia oil. It creates a long-lasting bacteria-killing barrier that stays intact even after washing and drying hands; it also provides the preventative hygiene that is so crucial in today's medical environments. Clearly, Anti-Bacterial Liquid Soap™ helps prevent the spread of disease and infection. For this reason alone, it should be advocated as standard fare, not only in every home, but also in every medical, dental and professional practice, too.

Many infections commonly seen today are caused by bacteria that have become highly resistant to being "knocked out" by antibiotics. In order to keep active, bacteria often changes its identity. For example, think of bacteria as a prize fighter that never stays on one side of the ring. It changes patterns, sometimes becoming the fighter and sometimes remaining the friend. But watch out! When least expected, it stands ready to deliver a knock-out punch to an opponent which, in this case, is the human body. Some suggest that even a nuclear blast will not knock down bacteria. Yet, Anti-Bacterial Liquid Soap™ comes the closest of any soap to eliminating bacteria. It is also the safest, longest-lasting and most concentrated antibacterial soap available to today's consumer market.

It soon became apparent that mentioning the general topic of infection meant going a few steps further and providing some basic, understandable information on the human body and the skin. Isn't it interesting that microbes living on skin can survive and thrive even in areas where complete sterilizing of the skin has been attempted? Scientists have learned that it is virtually impossible to create a site that will be perfectly microbe-free, since neither the air surrounding the site nor any surface becoming a contact point, can ever be completely sterilized.

In operating suites, bacteria can be reduced by pre-surgical scrubbing and by sterilizing the site, yet some patients develop severe allergic reactions to the sterilizers. This is one reason for the excitement about Melaleuca alternifolia oil in many medical, dental and veterinary situations. An increasing number of health care professionals are using Melaleuca alternifolia oil both before and after surgery. When the oil is used before surgery, post-operative infections often decrease and healing times are significantly reduced. Applied after surgery, the oil accelerates healing, reduces scarring and virtually eliminates the potential for developing secondary healing problems.

Researching information for this book led me to investigate how skin reacts when Melaleuca alternifolia oil is applied to it. In Minnesota, we could use an analogy for skin and refer to it as our down-filled jacket - it certainly is our protective wrap against cold weather, as well as being the body's largest organ!

A few years ago while at a business breakfast meeting, an acquaintance I had not seen for some time commented that I seemed to be putting on some extra weight. My defenses were "really elevated" that day. Without thinking, I told him I was on a special program with the University of Minnesota Medical School that was trying to figure out how far ordinary skin could actually stretch. . .

Healthy skin has the ability to resist injury and protect underlying tissues. The skin's principle function is to shield the internal organs from potential damage caused by outside forces, including the environment. The body's temperature is controlled by the skin. When the skin is hot, sweat glands shed perspiration. When the skin is cold, blood vessels constrict to conserve heat. The skin's outer layer makes "us" waterproof. For instance, this allows us to swim, without soaking up the water in which we are swimming. If the skin dries and becomes cracked, it provides an opportunity for any bacteria or infection to easily gain entry!

The epidermis is the skin's thin outside layer; it serves as a disposable covering. Beneath it is the dermis, a thick layer sometimes called the *true skin* because it contains most of the living elements. The epidermis contains cells that increase or decrease depending upon their exposure to external influences including injuries, the use of soaps and cosmetics, infections and other compromises to the immune system.

In the last ten years, the public has become increasingly aware of infections and viruses that depress the immune system. This can happen to anyone, of any age, race, life-style or ability who suffers from such well-known conditions as HIV or AIDS. Yet the world is filled with thousands of other viruses that also depress the body's immune system. One example of a virus-related condition appears to be acne. Those unfortunate enough to develop it are often forced to endure repeated outbreaks that can create permanent physical and lasting emotional scars.

Colds and flu are examples of other infections and viruses that can attack the human body. Regularly taking Melaleuca's Vitality Pak™ vitamins, drinking at least 8 to 10 glasses of water daily, drinking fruit juices rich in Vitamin C, and consuming numerous potfuls of G'Day™ Melaleuca Herbal Tea may well help avoid colds and flu. Using all of these will alleviate and treat many cold and flu symptoms after they've developed.

Hundreds and perhaps thousands of other viral conditions have unlimited opportunity to affect our lives. Drug companies have developed products that alleviate symptoms, although few if any, have introduced truly *breakthrough* drugs that cure or eliminate infections.

Scientists have discovered that many infections are **not** helped by synthetic drugs. Over a period of time, the bacteria can change and adapt to any medicine developed to fight it. When infections become drug-resistant they are almost impossible to eliminate with the use of drugs. Any virus immune to antibiotics can also become immune to antiseptics.

For the purposes of this book, I use the term "infection" as a broad catchall to include all infectious conditions. While some of these can be helped by antibiotics, others such as colds often become worse.

Dr. Merkert was our family doctor for many years. During the time I knew him, I learned his prescription for the common cold: Ten days, lots of fluids, plenty of rest and aspirin. Well, I believe that if the old Doc had stayed alive long enough, he would have come to know the therapeutic value of G'Day™ Melaleuca Herbal Tea. It's the only tea I know of that contains the healing leaves of the Melaleuca alternifolia tree. If it had been available four-plus decades ago, I'm convinced this doctor would have altered his treatment time to considerably less than ten days and probably dropped most of his other suggestions as well. However, I'll leave the discussion of colds and flu treatment suggestions to this book's later pages.

Today, everyone is susceptible to airborne infections. Nursing homes, hospitals and clinics are breeding grounds for antibiotic-resistant bacteria strains such as the common cold and influenza. Those with immune system deficiencies, including the very young and the elderly, are most susceptible to infections that "float around" in confined places. It stands to reason that the daily lack of fresh air is probably a culprit in the increasing numbers of people infected by airborne germs.

It only takes one look at a downtown high rise office building to realize that there are no open windows. The only air available is air that is exhaled and re-circulated through air filters that may be old or dirty. Is it clean air? That depends on your interpretation of the word "clean". My guess is that the air probably didn't pass by a clear river, grow bold in the woods or thin itself on a mountain range. We should ask ourselves: What actually is re-circulated air? And, where was our last breath before we inhaled it? We may well be surprised and disturbed with the answers we find to these questions.

After reading the above paragraphs, I don't want to give any reader the impression that all viruses are airborne. For example, AIDS cannot be transmitted by simply being in the presence of an infected person. It isn't spread by poor ventilation; no one has yet contracted the disease from breathing any re-circulated air.

As of mid-1995, the total number of American and Canadian lives infected by HIV and AIDS is estimated at well over 1.2 million; some 300,000 may have already died from these diseases.

The ages of those infected are represented by a cross-section between babies and the elderly. Perhaps the greatest number of deaths have occurred to people in their most productive years - their 20's, 30's and 40's. Behind each number stands a person - these aren't fence posts we're counting - each was once a viable living human being. We don't know how many were scientists, doctors, students, parents, engineers, elected or appointed officials, corporate leaders, inventors, writers and common-folk participants engaged in bettering their communities. We do know that each person who died represents a significant loss to a family, to a community and to our collective society as well.

Maybe this is a good place to urge you to visit the panels from the AIDS quilt if they ever come to your town. Plan to see them, or better yet take someone who's important to you, such as a child or grandchild. Walk with your family along the pathways between the rows of loss. It has been several years since I viewed the quilt, but one panel still haunts me with its words, *"There is no greater waste on earth than potential unrealized."*

Worldwide, an estimated 12 to 15 million people are infected by HIV and AIDS; this includes more than 1 million children. If a cure is not found and the disease is not stopped, it could claim 40 million women, children and men by the year 2000. *A good question to ask ourselves is - how many of these people will be from our own family, our own neighborhood. I urge you to think about your answer before you offer a quick response.*

The seriousness of the subject demands that any opportunity to discuss this nightmare should not be bypassed. That's why I'll borrow a slogan from a militant group that proclaims, "Silence equals death". This topic is too important to the health and well-being of us all to not mention it here. I don't believe there's ever a time when having too much knowledge will hurt anyone.

The reason I mention HIV and AIDS in a book such as this is simple. If we're to protect the lives of those we value and hold close, then we must by necessity educate them on the topics needed to survive in today's world. I urge each of you to learn as much as you can and pass along what you've learned with those who are important in your life.

I have come to realize that today's world is not the same world I was raised in. This one carries with it so many demands and potentially fatal pitfalls. While I would at times like to be 30 or 40 again - those times seem further apart when I consider the potential harm that comes with being younger. I don't think I would want to go through those years again, especially during these times. I'm thankful I've lived a good life, that I still have my mind somewhat intact (although some might argue this point), a sense of humor and a healthy outlook. I heard Johnny Carson, a television talk show host, once suggest that the secret of life is to die young - at a very old age. I absolutely agree.

People living with AIDS endure considerable problems with diseases of the skin, oral thrush and other conditions - some of which are described in this book. Melaleuca alternifolia oil and products containing the oil, are now used worldwide to alleviate some of the conditions and opportunistic infections that are associated with these diseases. However any treatment suggestion offered in these pages should be used only upon the approval of a physician or primary care-giver.

Hand-to-hand contact is the greatest factor contributing to the spread of infections. Grabbing handles and door knobs puts you in contact with bacteria. Then, when you rub your nose, or pick at a tooth (or vice-versa), harmful bacteria can enter your system. Washing your hands frequently is as important today as it was when your mother first told you about it. Hand washing is so basic that it is often overlooked as a practical method to prevent the spread of disease and infection.

Each of us must understand how Melaleuca alternifolia oil, and products containing the oil, can impact and affect our daily lives. Everyone must know how to routinely use these products. I know Melaleuca oil has helped me, just as I know the oil will help almost everyone who reads these words. It has improved my life and enhanced my well-being, and based upon that, I am everlastingly confident it can do the same for the majority of those reading this. It is because of my personal experience that I recommend that nearly everyone (subject to cautions printed throughout these pages) can confidently use Melaleuca oil. Consider it something you're doing to help yourself. Make a personal decision and commitment to use products containing Melaleuca alternifolia oil - if only for the health of it!

Introduction To
Personal Care Facts

The preceding pages have explained a brief history of the development of Melaleuca alternifolia oil. I refer to all that precedes these words as "introduction-fodder" for the Personal Care Facts presented in this section. I want to emphasize again some important precautionary statements. Please consider them your personal reminder to become a student and learn to "know thyself" before attempting any new or newly suggested treatment ideas using any new products.

In the pages that follow, I frequently use the words, "Suggested Treatment". Several readers have inquired as to how I can suggest a treatment when I'm not a doctor or a specially trained medical professional. I have freely stated throughout these pages that I am neither. *I do however freely admit to being a writer and a mortal; hopefully, I won't be challenged on these two claims.*

I took these comments seriously and considered replacement phrases that might be appropriate. However, I found that nothing really worked as well as "Suggested Treatment".

It was at this point that I decided to use *Webster's Third New International Dictionary* to obtain accurate definitions for the words "suggest" and "treatment". *"**Suggest**" is defined as, "... to put (as an idea, proposition, or impulse) into the mind ... to mention (something) as a possibility ... to propose (something) as desirable or fitting ... to offer (as an idea or theory) for consideration."* And, *"**Treatment**" is defined as, "... The action or manner of treating [a person] medically ... the action or manner of dealing with something in a specified way ... preventative guidance ..."*

Combining the two words, then, means mentioning something as a possibility and dealing with something in a specified way. To my way of thinking, this just shows that even common folk can offer a suggested treatment using ordinary language and understandable syntax. *("Syntax" is defined as, "the arrangement of word forms to show their mutual relations in the sentence".) Well, I had the book open and couldn't resist looking up this word, too.*

Please understand that any product use or suggested treatment mentioned in these pages should not be considered a substitute for obtaining appropriate medical treatment from a physician or primary care-giver. If you have a medical problem, condition or illness, always consult your physician or primary care-giver well *before* beginning any new program or treatment. Do NOT alter any prescribed medication or treatment before consultation with your physician or primary care-giver when and where needed.

Do you go to a health-care doctor or a medical doctor? There is a difference. Health-care doctors dispense health-care information, discuss possible remedies or alternative therapies and offer advice on a whole spectrum of potential treatments. Medical doctors practice medicine. To me, the word "practice" has always seemed an interesting word choice when considering that this is the professional to whom most of us trust our lives and hopes for a long future. Personally, I'd feel much better if they didn't refer to what they did each day as practice ... Maybe this is the reason why I now expect my doctor to be a health-care professional.

Products containing Melaleuca alternifolia oil generally work well on almost everyone. However, there are exceptions. **People with contact dermatitis should not use the pure oil.** Those allergic to fragrances should read product labels carefully and use only those products that are fragrance-free; some Melaleuca products do contain fragrances.

Knowing yourself and being aware of possible or potential problems before they happen is your safest assurance of maintaining good health. It is important to remember that Melaleuca alternifolia oil-based products, as with any products, are not universal cure-alls that will work in the same manner for everyone. Determining proper choices for personal care, health and well-being, will help you enhance your life. Remember: If you do nothing, you also are making a choice.

The following pages list a variety of conditions and suggest ideas for treatment. This listing is incomplete. If you know of other conditions that respond to Melaleuca alternifolia oil or products containing the oil, I would like to know about them. Future editions will hopefully contain additional data and testimonials. Your comments and suggestions are important.

PERSONAL CARE FACTS

Please Note: The listing of Personal Care Facts that follows is far from complete. If you know of other conditions that respond favorably to this oil, or products containing the oil, why not tell us so we can inform other readers about what's worked best for you? The more facts we have, the better we can deal with the calamities and day-to-day problems associated with ordinary living. Having too much knowledge is never a problem when it comes to addressing how to best manage our personal care and that of our families. Remember, there's a personally autographed S.T. Clark™ book waiting for you if your suggestion is the first like it that's received; so…?

ABRASIONS

Scrapes and cuts that break the skin's surface. When injured, the immediate area can become red and inflamed. White blood cells that fight infection rush to the site. As healing begins, scabs form natural bandages that protect the injured area.

Suggested Treatment: Wash with Anti-Bacterial Liquid Soap™ and warm water. Pat dry and apply T36-C7™. As this dries, apply Problem Skin Lotion™, Mela-Gel™ or Triple Antibiotic Ointment™. Your choice will depend on preference and the type or location of the injury. Infection is less likely to develop if you use this treatment as soon as an injury occurs. If you are somewhere where you cannot easily clean the abrasion, apply T36-C7™ even without washing. An area injured can always be subsequently cleaned. Eliminating the risk of infection is the immediate concern.

Note: Tetanus can occur when abrasions are deep or contaminated. If it has been more than five years since your tetanus shot, immediately contact your physician or health-care provider. People who die from tetanus are generally older adults who are not current on their booster shots.

ACNE (PIMPLES AND BLACKHEADS)

This condition primarily affects adolescents and can occur on almost any part of the body. Outbreaks generally appear on the face, chest and upper back. Factors believed to contribute to acne outbreaks include diet, hormonal changes and bacterial infection of the sebaceous glands. One contributing cause also appears related to exposure to oil and grease, where extended periods of contact with cooking oil, such as in restaurant kitchens, can make outbreaks worse. Additional factors can include the use of oil-based cosmetics, the use of some prescription drugs, heredity (where the condition often seems to "run" in some families) and changes in the human body at the onset of puberty.

Acne also affects adults under stress; outbreaks will often occur in women during pregnancy. Despite what some written accounts have previously "verified", it appears to be mostly a myth that eating chocolate or consuming a particular food will cause or aggravate acne outbreaks. While proper hygiene, including at least twice daily washing of areas most prone to becoming affected, will not in and of itself prevent acne, it may well help to reduce or limit the natural spreading inherent in most acne outbreaks.

Suggested Treatment: At least twice daily, usually in the morning and the evening, wash the affected area(s) thoroughly using Anti-Bacterial Liquid Soap™ or the Gold Bar™. Apply Zap-It™ as directed on the product label. Follow with applications of T36-C7™ every two hours. After healing begins, apply T36-C7™ followed by Problem Skin Lotion™. John suggests using this as an alternative treatment: After applying Zap-It™ and obtaining preliminary relief, follow with Impressions™ Skin Nurturing System products; use according to directions and in conjunction with the Gold Bar™. John asked me to be sure to mention that Zap-It™ should be applied **only** to the specific acne and definitely not as an all-over facial or body creme.

ALLERGIC RASHES

Begin as the immune system's negative reaction to a third-party influence such as that caused by exposure to chemicals, pollen, dust particles, a particular food, or other irritant. Allergic rashes are often accompanied by itching, redness and sometimes by a type of overall body soreness that appears in flu-like symptoms.

Suggested Treatment: Products such as T36-C7™, Body Satin™ Lotion or Problem Skin Lotion™ will help alleviate the pain and itching caused by most allergic rashes. If the rash is severe, use Mela-Gel™. Ted's wife Mary suggests adding 1 capful Natural Spa & Bath Oil™ to a tub of warm water. It helps alleviate the discomfort of an allergic rash and is a perfect way to "wind down" after a busy day. After soaking, gently dry the rash area and apply T36-C7™ followed by a Melaleuca lotion of your choice.

ARTHRITIS

Inflammation of the joints frequently accompanied by swelling, skin redness and painful impaired motion. Osteoarthritis, the most common form is chronic and afflicts millions. It can involve the hands, shoulders, knees, hips and spine. Rheumatoid arthritis is a chronic systemic disease characterized by inflammatory changes in the joints that often result in painful crippling.

Suggested Treatment: Very gently massage affected areas with T36-C7™.

Follow with Pain-A-Trate™. Using these in sequence and in frequent applications will help reduce swelling and may eliminate most associated pain. Many suffering from arthritis have written to tell me how they found particular relief when they applied Melaleuca products. Others claim they have been significantly helped by regularly taking Mel-Vita™ and Mela-Cal™ vitamins and by drinking several potfuls daily of G'Day™ Melaleuca Herbal Tea.

ATHLETE'S FOOT

Usually caused by a fungal infection. Outbreaks generally occur between the toes where the skin has a greater tendency to crack, become blistered or sore and itchy. While this is generally the most common area affected, the condition sometimes appears on the scalp and extremities, too. Athlete's Foot is commonly found in athletic showering areas; yet many suffering from it could never be confused with being athletic. However, Athlete's Foot rarely develops in young children or in those who generally go barefoot or wear sandals.

Suggested Treatment: Clean affected areas with Anti-Bacterial Liquid Soap™. Rinse well with water. Dry thoroughly and apply T36-C7™. Lightly coat the affected area with Problem Skin Lotion™ or Mela-Gel™. Repeat the process morning and evening. Richard recommends continuing the treatments for at least a week following the condition clearing to assure that it has been fully healed.

For stubborn or persistent infections, soak the affected area for 20 minutes. To warm water, add 1 teaspoonful Sol-U-Mel™ and 1 teaspoonful Natural Spa & Bath Oil™. Repeat this procedure at least twice daily for 7-10 days. Greg, the most completely athletic person I know, uses an old ice chest for foot soaking. He claims that since the chest seals in the cold, it should also keep the water warmer than using a pan or tub.

This may sound more like your mother talking, but if your outbreak is actually on your feet, change your socks and footwear daily. Some find extra relief when lightly spraying the insides of their shoes with a mixture of 1 part Sol-U-Mel™ with 10 parts water. I would suggest adding several drops of T36-C7™ to this mixture, too.

BED SORES

Affect people confined to one place for long periods of time. When considering bed sores, I think first of the elderly, stroke patients, and those with life-threatening or terminal illnesses.

Suggested Treatment: Gently clean the sores and surrounding area using either the Gold Bar™ or Anti-Bacterial Liquid Soap™. Pat dry and apply T36-C7™. The oil will penetrate deeply to heal injured tissue. Lightly coat all skin areas that are distressed, since they are often the primary pressure points between the patient and the bed.

Problem Skin Lotion™ and Mela-Gel™ help repair and hydrate damaged skin areas. Body Satin™ Lotion or Melaleuca Hand Creme™ should be applied several times daily. Be sure to also coat those areas most prone to developing additional sores.

It's important to couple treatment with preventative actions that will help prevent future bed sores from forming. Minimizing pressure on areas prone to develop sores is crucial. Placing pillows, cushions and ripple types of pressurized mattresses under the patient will help decrease the chances of the patient developing future sores; sheepskin wraps for the heels and buttocks may also be helpful. A growing list of long-term care-staffs are now using Melaleuca alternifolia oil and products containing the oil, having discovered the oil's effectiveness in accelerating healing and alleviating patient discomfort.

BEE STINGS

Usually stings are immediately painful, yet sometimes they are actually beneficial. I know about the beneficial aspect since a bee sting prompted my introduction to Melaleuca alternifolia oil. Bee stings cause an immediate "surprise" pain. The site of the sting will become red and very sore.

Suggested Treatment: Be sure to inspect the bite area to determine if the stinger is still in the skin. If possible, remove it carefully without squeezing to avoid breaking the venom sack. For best results, apply T36-C7™ liberally to the site. As the oil starts to dry, liberally apply Mela-Gel™. Repeat applications 4 to 6 times - applying T36-C7™ first, followed by Mela-Gel™; repeat every half hour over a 2 to 3 hour period. Thereafter, follow this same process as often as needed. *(Maybe it was an old bee that first stung me in that strawberry patch in Southeastern Minnesota, since the stinging pain disappeared after just one application of T36-C7™.)*

Remember: If you are allergic to bee stings, it is important to your health AND LIFE to follow the directions in your antidote kit. Immediately seek the nearest medical assistance. Bee stings can be life-threatening.

BLEEDING GUMS

Often caused by an inflammation, mild cases are commonly seen in pregnant women and in diabetics, both of whom experience significant changes in hormone levels. Young adults often appear to have more mild cases.

Bleeding gums can often be alleviated by adopting a regular routine of good oral hygiene that includes brushing teeth at least twice daily with the proper tooth polish. Careful brushing that avoids raking or tearing at sensitive gum tissues, is essential in preventing bleeding gums. Many claim that by using Melaleuca's Tooth Polish, flossing daily with Denti-Care System™ Dental Tape and frequent gargling with Breath-Away™ Mouth Wash, they have eliminated bleeding gums. In addition, I would also regularly take Mel-Vita™ and Mela-Cal™ vitamins (*I take two of each both morning and evening with meals*), drinking at least 8 to 10 glasses of water daily and maintaining a diet of healthier foods.

Suggested Treatment: Using your finger tip or cotton swab, apply T36-C7™ to affected gums. Most people do not enjoy the taste of pure Melaleuca alternifolia oil. However, I don't know of anyone who has applied the oil to their bleeding gums who hasn't later extolled the healing virtues of Melaleuca alternifolia oil. There is a lesson or two to be learned here. A product doesn't have to taste good, or sweet, to accomplish healing. A *Melaleuca-mouth* is far better than one harboring sore or bleeding gums.

BLISTERS

Oval-shaped raised areas of skin holding collections of fluid beneath the outer layer of skin. They are frequently caused by friction or burns such as sunburn. Blisters can also be caused by skin conditions such as eczema, impetigo and dermatitis. Sometimes, they occur when an area is scratched repeatedly. Blisters should not be punctured.

Suggested Treatment: I know from personal experience that blisters diminish after *gingerly* applying T36-C7™. Dab the oil on the blistered area, then leave alone until the next application. When I use Melaleuca oil, my blisters heal over quickly without itching or burning.

BODY MASSAGE

This is not a condition as much as it is a preferred treatment. It is a truly wonderful remedy for easing life's aches and pains.

Suggested Treatment: Why not follow Nancy's suggestion? She reports "absolutely wonderful results" mixing a bottle of liquid Pain-A-Trate™ with a bottle of Body Satin™ Lotion. *I have tried her suggestion and now agree that it makes a "rub" seem right. See if you don't agree. Why not rub a favorite body sometime soon?*

BODY ODOR

Well friends, this should be relatively easy for most everyone to figure out. Maybe it's so easy that it should not be listed here. Then again, if you are around someone who has body odor, you have to wonder why they do not notice it, too.

Suggested Treatment: Start by giving the offensive person a Gold Bar™. Tell them how well it works for you and how effectively it can work for them.

Encourage them to use Melaleuca's Herbal Shampoo™. If you've reached this point in the conversation and are still standing, gently explain that after they shower or bathe, they should use At-Last™ Antiperspirant Deodorant. Tell them how it will help them smell better - longer, enjoy more friendships and have more friends who'll enjoy their friendship and companionship.

Notwithstanding my feeble attempts at a humorous suggestion, body odor can sometimes be a body's first warning signal of significant medical problems. If the suggested treatments outlined above don't work, the person with this problem, should consult with their physician or primary care-giver for an in-depth check-up or physical exam to determine the cause of their b.o.

BOILS

A painful red swelling in the skin caused by a bacterial infection of a hair follicle or sweat gland. Boils generally appear on the neck, breast, face and buttocks.

Suggested Treatment: Clean the area affected with Anti-Bacterial Liquid Soap™. Then apply T36-C7™ several times daily. Follow with Problem Skin Lotion™. If aggressive treatment is indicated, follow these suggestions every 2 to 3 hours daily for approximately 7 to 10 days.

Some recommend hot soaks, adding 1 to 2 tablespoonfuls Natural Spa & Bath Oil™ to a quart of warm water. Dampen a cloth in the solution and place it over the boil. Keep the boil covered for 10 minutes. Repeat as necessary.

BROMHIDROSIS

Excessively sweaty feet can occur in people of all ages. While it is often attributed to nervousness, it can also be caused by other factors. If it can't be readily eliminated by the suggested treatments, you should consult with your physician or primary care-giver.

Suggested Treatment: Use the Gold Bar™ or Anti-Bacterial Liquid Soap™ to wash the feet well, including the areas between the toes. Rinse and pat dry. Apply T36-C7™ to the soles of the feet and between the toes. Repeat this process at least twice daily. Change socks after each application to help eliminate odor.

BRONCHITIS

An inflammation of the major airways branching from the windpipe and leading into the lungs. Bronchial inflammation is typically aggravated by environmental pollutants including cigarette smoke, dust and chemical vapors.

Suggested Treatment: Drink at least 7 to 10 glasses of water daily. Avoid forced air heat and over-the-counter medicines that dry coughs, suppressing the beneficial coughing action that brings up phlegm. Add 1 tablespoonful

Sol-U-Mel™ and 5 to 10 drops T36-C7™ in a vaporizer filled with water. Make a "tent" by draping a large towel (such as a bath or even a beach towel) over both your head and the vaporizer. Breathe the vapors for 10 minutes. Repeat this process at least twice daily. Many people find additional relief when sleeping in a room with a vaporizer or cold mist humidifier. Be sure to add Sol-U-Mel™ and T36-C7™ to the tank's water.

Note: Consult your regular physician or primary care-giver if any of these conditions are present: Fever, intensified attacks or coughing up blood. A physician or primary care-giver should always be consulted if the person suffering from bronchitis has other underlying medical or lung problems.

BUNIONS

Firm fluid-filled pads that form on the joint at the base of the big toe. When inflamed, they can be very painful.

Suggested Treatment: My Aunt Cora advocates adding 1 tablespoonful Sol-U-Mel™ in a quart (or so) of warm water for a foot soak and soaking the foot for 10 to 15 minutes. After drying, apply T36-C7™ and MelaGel™ or Problem Skin Lotion™. Commercial toe pads also will help if the bunion is small. Aunt Cora suggests that doing something as simple as wearing proper fitting shoes is important in preventing future bunions. A caution to this suggestion is that if you have large or recurring bunions, your physician or primary care-giver should be consulted prior to initiating self-treatment. Bunions will, if not treated or if treated incorrectly or infrequently, usually get worse and ultimately may even require corrective surgery in order to eliminate.

BURNS

Each year more than 2,000,000 Americans are burned or scalded severely enough to obtain medical treatment. Of these, some 70,000 require hospitalization. The majority of burn victims are children and the elderly. Accidents at home account for most burns. It is important to recognize the type of burn injury incurred. For example, first-degree burns such as sunburn cause reddening and generally affect only the top layer of skin. These burns should heal quickly. Second-degree burns usually heal without scarring, unless they are extensive and cover a larger area. Third-degree burns destroy the skin's full thickness, leaving the surface looking white or even charred. These burns usually require special treatment and frequently need skin grafts to prevent scarring. Electrical burns show little surface damage, yet cause internal destruction including damage to the heart. First-degree burns cause pain. Second and third-degree burns cause pain and shock. They may be fatal if left untreated. Third-degree burns and electrical burns require immediate professional medical treatment.

Suggested Treatment: Burn experts recommend flushing the burn immediately with ice cold water. For minor burns, carefully pat dry and apply T36-C7™. Cover the burned area gently with Problem Skin Lotion™. Repeat this process two or three times daily until tissues are healed. If the skin blisters, or is somewhat charred, loosely cover with sterile gauze. Change the gauze daily.

Several restaurant owners I know, keep bottles of T36-C7™ on hand for treating grill and fryer burns. Melaleuca alternifolia oil is non-toxic and provides an anesthetic-like action. It soothes and alleviates most pain on contact. It also will help prevent blistering and even scarring. Since infections nearly always develop in severe burns, frequent applications of T36-C7™ will help stop itching and accelerate healing.

CANKER SORES

Mouth ulcers that appear on the lips and inside the mouth. They are extremely painful, particularly for those who, like myself, wear dentures. Even a small sore becomes the permanent raspberry seed under a plate (or denture). Those with their own teeth probably cannot imagine this. So, compare it to walking around with a permanent nail in the bottom of your shoe. When mature, the sores usually display a white tip that is filled with fluid or pus. Sores can be caused by eating too many nuts and citrus fruits. They also can be attributed to a deficiency of essential amino acids.

Suggested Treatment: When a canker sore first appears, dab T36-C7™ on your finger and apply to the sore at least once every few hours. Usually after a few applications, the sore will *go away*. However, sometimes sores may take several days to heal.

I have had fewer canker sores since switching to Melaleuca's Denti-Care System™, using Hot Shot™ Breath & Throat Spray, Melaleuca's Tooth Polish and Breath-Away™ Mouth Wash. I generally use a mixture of 1 part Mouth Wash to 8 parts water. When I have a canker sore, I will use a mixture twice as strong. I also "enjoy" the feeling that Melaleuca's Tooth Polish gives my mouth. I just load my plate with it before returning the denture to my mouth. *This is one instance where loading your plate will really help you.*

CARBUNCLES

Clusters of boils having deep infections that cover large skin areas. Generally carbuncles are slow to develop. This allows aggressive treatment to be initiated before the carbuncle is mature. Sometimes carbuncles are accompanied by fever. While diabetes and old age are often contributing factors, anyone can develop carbuncles.

Suggested Treatment: Clean the affected area with Anti-Bacterial Liquid Soap™. When dry, apply T36-C7™ followed by Problem Skin Lotion™.

Repeat this process several times daily. If aggressive treatment is needed, follow these suggestions every 2 to 3 hours during the day. This aggressive treatment schedule should be used no longer than 7 to 10 days. Some recommend hot tub soaks (if the carbuncle is where it can be soaked). Use 1 to 2 tablespoonfuls Natural Spa & Bath Oil™ in a tub of warm water. Otherwise, dampen a cloth in the solution and cover the carbuncle for 10 to 15 minutes. Pat dry and apply T36-C7™ followed by Problem Skin Lotion™.

CHAPPED HANDS

Often caused by excessive exposure to cleaners, solvents, detergents and soapy water. This condition is characterized by small cuts or cracks in the skin.

Suggested Treatment: Wash hands thoroughly with Anti-Bacterial Liquid Soap™, then dry well. Apply T36-C7™ to any severely chapped areas, cover with either Problem Skin Lotion™ or Hand Creme™. Massage well into skin. If skin cracks still appear, repeat this cycle of washing before drying then apply the pure Melaleuca alternifolia oil with a covering lotion or cream. Be sure to repeat this procedure several times throughout the day. *By regularly using Body Satin™ Lotion, my hands remain moist - but not sticky - throughout the day. I also use Hand Creme™ to alleviate my chapped hands and dry skin.*

CHAPPED LIPS

Apply either the vanilla or pina colada Sun-Shades™ Lip Balm. *If I were forced to choose between the flavors, I would take the pina colada, because frankly being Norwegian, I have enough things that are bland and vanilla.* However, either flavor is excellent.

CHICKEN POX

Generally affects children and young adults. The rash develops from pink, flat spots into tiny, single blisters that become dry and encrusted within 2 to 4 days. The rash often itches severely. Scratching should be avoided because it can lead to bacterial infection of the skin and the subsequent formation of scars.

Suggested Treatment: Wash the affected area with Anti-Bacterial Liquid Soap™. Pat dry and liberally apply T36-C7™. Allow the oil sufficient time to soak into the skin. Later, add 2 capfuls Natural Spa & Bath Oil™ in a tub of warm water. After soaking affected areas for 10 to 15 minutes, gingerly pat dry and reapply T36-C7™. When the oil has started absorbing into the skin, or is drying, apply either Mela-Gel™ or Problem Skin Lotion™. Repeat this process at least several times throughout the day. **As with every suggestion contained in these pages, if complications develop, if symptoms worsen, or if there's no improvement within a reasonable time, absolutely contact your physician or primary care-giver.**

CHIGGERS

There is nothing like a walk through the meadow on a summer afternoon. Then again, there is nothing quite like the itch from a chigger eruption on your feet, legs and thighs caused by that stroll. Mite infestations are more frequent in the southern regions of the country than here in the Upper Midwest. Wherever they are, mites cause chiggers which can cause you to rush to use this treatment.

Suggested Treatment: Cleanse the affected area with Anti-Bacterial Liquid Soap™. After drying, apply T36-C7™ followed by Problem Skin Lotion™ or Mela-Gel™. Repeat this process morning and evening. Anne's chigger recipe calls for combining 1 capful Natural Spa & Bath Oil™, 1 capful Sol-U-Mel™ and 2-3 pumps Anti-Bacterial Liquid Soap™ in a quart of warm water. Soak the affected or bitten areas for at least 15 minutes using a wet cloth. Pat dry before applying T36-C7™, followed by Problem Skin Lotion™ or Mela-Gel™.

COLD SORES

Caused by the herpes simplex virus. Outbreaks affect all age brackets including infants, children and adults. Cold sores are characterized by clear fluid-filled eruptions that appear on the lips and inside the mouth. Some factors that may contribute to outbreaks include menstruation, fever, food allergies or toothbrush abrasions.

Symptoms generally last less than ten days. Sometimes cold sores are so painful that it becomes difficult to chew foods and swallow liquids. Those having secondary health problems where intake of food and liquid are essential (such as seniors, very young children, diabetics, or those with low blood sugar) need to be particularly careful that their cold sores don't interfere with any other medical problems they may be experiencing.

Suggested Treatment: Immediately apply T36-C7™ to the sores at the first sign of a lesion or probable outbreak. The primary goal in aggressive cold sore treatment is to recognize sores before they come to a head, and to then initiate immediate treatment. Apply T36-C7™ and Mela-Gel™ at least every 2 hours. For sores inside the mouth, gargle with 10 drops T36-C7™ blended with a half-cupful warm water. Repeat several times daily. Dab T36-C7™ onto your finger or a cotton swab and apply to the affected area. Regularly use Breath-Away™ Mouth Wash, Melaleuca's Tooth Polish and Hot Shot™ Mouth & Throat Spray.

CONGESTION

Can indicate the onset of a cold or an allergic reaction.

Suggested Treatment: Try rubbing T36-C7™ followed by Body Satin™ Lotion on your upper chest and around the throat. Dab T36-C7™ beneath each nostril to breathe easier and help clear nasal congestion. Adding 8-10 drops T36-C7™ and 1 capful Sol-U-Mel™ to a vaporizer also helps. If no relief is obtained, or if the condition persists or deteriorates, contact your physician or primary care-giver. If there is no apparent reason for the congestion, allergy tests may help to determine the exact cause.

CORAL CUTS

Left untreated or treated incorrectly, coral cuts may be serious and lead to infection. Some form of aggressive treatment should always be initiated whenever any coral cuts have been incurred.

Suggested Treatment: Thoroughly and gently clean all cuts with Anti-Bacterial Liquid Soap™. Pat dry and apply T36-C7™ followed by Triple Antibiotic Ointment™. Continue treatment every 2 to 3 hours until the cuts start healing and form protective scabs.

CORNS

A painful, localized thickening of the skin on the foot. Corns are caused by friction or pressure. Soft corns usually occur in protected areas such as between the toes. Hard corns appear on the tops, bottoms and sides of the feet. Corns sometimes ache, become tender and may be sensitive to pressure.

Suggested Treatment: Add 1 tablespoonful Sol-U-Mel™ to a quart of warm water and soak the foot for 15 minutes. Dry thoroughly and apply T36-C7™ followed by Mela-Gel™ or Problem Skin Lotion™. Repeating this procedure several times daily for a few days should soften the corn enough so it can be easily (and painlessly) removed with a tweezer.

Diabetics who frequently suffer from poor foot circulation and healing problems should first consult with their physician or primary care-giver before initiating the above suggested treatment.

COUGHS

Usually caused by an irritant such as exposure to smoke, dust or environmental pollutants, or something more common such as a cold or build-up of throat mucus. Coughs can also be another one of the body's early warning signals; persistent coughs may indicate a potentially serious medical problem. If coughing continues for longer than several days or a week, and no improvement is noted, contact your physician or primary care-giver. If coughing is caused by a common irritant, by the flu or cold, the following may help alleviate symptoms.

Suggested Treatment: Apply T36-C7™ followed by Body Satin™ Lotion on your upper chest and around your throat. Dab T36-C7™ under each nostril as this will help you breathe easier. When I have a problem with coughing, I park a vaporizer by my bed each night and add 10-12 drops T36-C7™ to the water tank and at least 1 to 2 capfuls Sol-U-Mel. **Absolutely do not ignore any cough that is unresponsive to treatment. Seek professional advice from a physician or primary care-giver if symptoms persist, particularly if the "cougher" has other medical problems.**

CRADLE CAP

May develop in infants usually during their first month of life. While we do not have any babies in our home now, I do have new-parent friends who have used the following treatment and suggest it may work for others, too.

Suggested Treatment: Make a very diluted mixture of T36-C7™ blended with olive oil. Combine thoroughly and apply to affected area. Leave on for several minutes before shampooing with a Melaleuca shampoo.

CUTS

Narrow slices or slashes that break the skin's surface. When skin is cut, the immediate area becomes red and inflamed. White blood cells which fight infection rush to the site. As cuts heal, scabs form natural bandages that protect the injured site.

Suggested Treatment: Clean with Anti-Bacterial Liquid Soap™ and warm water. Pat dry and apply T36-C7™. Follow with Problem Skin Lotion™, Mela-Gel™ or Triple Antibiotic Ointment™. Cuts heal faster and have less opportunity to develop infections if this treatment is used as soon as an injury occurs.

If you are somewhere where you cannot easily clean the cut, immediately apply T36-C7™. Melaleuca alternifolia oil will penetrate deeply into the injured skin to begin healing. Any injured area can always be cleaned. The primary concern is to initiate a treatment that will help eliminate future infections.

Note: Tetanus can occur when cuts are deep or contaminated. If it has been more than five years since your last tetanus shot, immediately contact your physician or primary care-giver. The majority of victims dying from tetanus are older adults who have not kept current on their booster shots.

DANDRUFF

A common scalp problem that primarily affects adults. At one time, it was believed that dandruff was caused by poor personal hygiene. Sometimes it is an indication of unusually dry skin. Home remedies usually consist of trying to increase the scalp's oil. Usually this only results in creating more dandruff.

Many dermatologists believe that dandruff is another form (albeit a mild one) of seborrheic dermatitis, which can be caused by a yeast-like fungus. Seborrheic dermatitis is an inflammation of the skin that can appear on the scalp and eyebrows. It is characterized by flaky white scaly skin that sloughs off, leaving a dry or greasy scalp that produces the itching so common with dandruff.

There are others who believe dandruff is caused by using harsh detergents, soaps and chemical-laden shampoos that challenge normal skin bacteria. Other factors may include stress and poor diet.

Suggested Treatment: Frequently, at least one or two times daily, shampoo with Melaleuca's Natural Shampoo™. It contains an abundance of healing Melaleuca oil and works particularly well to treat almost any type of common scalp condition including dandruff. Since this shampoo contains conditioner, no extra conditioner that could possibly be a scalp irritant, should be used. I think you'll find that Melaleuca's Natural Shampoo™ will really clean and invigorate your hair.

*I don't like going through my day with my hair smelling like another person's perfume. Call me old fashioned if you like, but I just can't get use to anything that forces me to smell like something some chemist somewhere thought I might like to smell like. This statement brings me to telling you what I really appreciate about Melaleuca's Natural Shampoo™. It doesn't carry with it any extra baggage such as a lingering perfume or even a vague chemical odor. Plus, it's extremely concentrated, which would have been real important - even if it **had** smelled - to some of my ancestors. I say that with tongue-in-cheek because as I get older and more frugal, saving money by buying products with low-cost-per-use factors is becoming important to me. One bottle of Melaleuca's shampoo lasts me well over a month of my daily use. If you're already a Melaleuca customer, you know what I'm referring to!*

Melaleuca affords me the luxury of saving money while shopping from the comforts of home. I find it relaxing looking out across a frozen lake, sitting by a crackling fire, or listening to Bach and enjoying a glass (or two) of wine. When I'm ready to shop, I just pick up the telephone to order a supply of shampoo, soap, vitamins and all the other personal and home-care products we routinely purchase each month from Melaleuca. I don't have to venture out into the below zero wind-chills of February or lug supplies in from the car, or try to find a cool place in the August heat to shop at. Plus, my checkbook is far quieter with all the price savings routinely available when buying Melaleuca's concentrated products!

*To those who don't know what I'm referring to, maybe it's time to put down this book and pick up the phone. Call someone who can show you how easy it is to become a preferred customer. That's another thing I like about Melaleuca - I'm preferred - not just a cog in a wheel, a circle or square on a scrap of paper, a dot on a growth chart. **At Melaleuca, I'm special - and I'm preferred!***

DENTAL DECAY

Heredity is a factor in tooth decay. *My father's teeth were soft and he wore dentures as long as I knew him. By the time I was 20, I had "store-bought" teeth. I always thought that teeth should last when your diet included lutefisk, lefse, potatoes and dairy products, but these fine Scandinavian treats didn't prevent my tooth decay and tooth loss.*

When I was young, good dental care meant brushing daily. Now, we're told that we should brush after each meal and floss daily. To avoid the problems I experienced years ago, follow good dental hygiene by visiting your dentist regularly and using Melaleuca's Denti-Care System™.

Maintaining healthy teeth includes removing plaque before it calcifies and turns into a tartar that cannot be removed with a toothbrush. Tartar forms along the gum line where it encourages stains and tooth decay. It can be removed by brushing, but when it adheres to the rough surfaces, it is almost impossible to eliminate by brushing. Untreated, plaque can lead to inflammation and periodontal disease.

The American Dental Association reports that three out of every four adults suffer from some form of gum disease. Bacterial plaque is the cause of tooth loss and infection. Melaleuca's Dental Tape™ is unique since it contains T36-C7™. This tape is flat rather than spherical. Plus it is strong and won't break like other dental flosses when used between closely spaced teeth. People who routinely use this cinnamon flavored tape claim that after flossing, their mouths feel so "satisfied" they want to sit back and relax in the enjoyment of the moment. *Ted mentions that when he uses Melaleuca's Dental Tape™, his mouth undergoes a near-spiritual experience.*

Prior to a dental appointment, Mindy dabs a few drops of T36-C7™ on her gums. She claims this helps reduce infection and pain from any dental treatments. Following the appointment, she applies T36-C7™ for added relief. If a tooth is extracted, T36-C7™ applied to the site will help accelerate healing. While it doesn't taste particularly good, it does taste like it must be working. *The only advantage I can tell you about having store-bought teeth is that now when I go to the dentist's office, I sit and hold onto the chair's side rails as the dentist grinds away on my teeth - in the next room. You can call me old-fashioned, but I still shiver and I am still nervous.*

Suggested Treatment: Many, including this writer, suggest at least daily use of each product in Melaleuca's Dental Care System™. This includes Melaleuca's Tooth Polish, Breath-Away™ Mouth Wash, and the Dental Care™ System Dental Tape™. I know that by using T36-C7™ and almost any product containing Melaleuca alternifolia oil, gum or tooth soreness and pain can be eliminated. It just makes real good sense for those who still have their own teeth to take particularly good care of them. If you're diabetic or have another condition where regular diet and regular food consumption are critical to maintaining your good health, you don't need me to remind you how important it is that your teeth and mouth are healthy and working properly.

As someone who's living life fully but without his own teeth, I urge you to do all you can to avoid dental decay. In retrospect, I wish now that I had been more watchful, observant and knowledgeable about dental decay - particularly, while I still had the opportunity to do something about it. This is my excuse, but, what's yours? Its never too late to start using a system that can really help. But the clock is ticking, and the time is now. So the next move - or removal - is really up to you!

DERMATITIS

Inflammation of the skin caused by an outside irritant that can produce itchy, red skin. It will, when irritated and scratched, produce small blisters. Acute types of dermatitis can be characterized by red, blistered and swollen areas. In chronic stages, dermatitis is evidenced by dry, scaly and thickened skin patches.

Suggested Treatment: Cleanse affected areas with Anti-Bacterial Liquid Soap™. Pat dry and follow with Problem Skin Lotion™. CAUTION: Avoid using the pure oil to treat any dermatitis condition. Dermatitis is often caused by reactions to chemical exposure and harsh detergents. (Refer to *"Home Safety Facts."*)

DIABETES & DIABETIC FOOT ULCERATIONS

Ulcerations frequently occur in those who are over the age of 40 and have had diabetes for more than 10 years. Other contributing factors include: obesity, lack of exercise and improper care of the feet. Diabetes causes blood vessel walls to thicken. This decreases the blood flow to the feet and lower legs.

Diabetes causes damage to the foot and leg nerves (a condition called "neuropathy"). Nerves act as the body's alarm that realizes or senses pain, temperature and pressure. Neuropathy makes feet numb, unable to feel heat, cold, pressure, cuts or bruises. Some diabetics suffer from neuropathy *and* poor circulation. These conditions can combine to create a situation where even *routine* cuts, blisters and scrapes can develop into gangrene. If not treated aggressively, gangrene will result in limb amputation.

Since being diagnosed as diabetic some three years ago, I continue to inject insulin twice daily. I have, during this time, experienced foot problems that I can thankfully still call "minor". Melaleuca's products have been VERY effective in treating all of them. I can personally attest to the value of these products in my own diabetic care program.

Every morning I take vitamins from Melaleuca's Vitality Pak™, finding that since they're fructose compounded, they're disguised as a sugar and can enter my blood stream quickly. I also regularly take Cell-Wise® and

ProVex™ Super-Antioxidants, finding that not only do I feel healthier and more energetic, but I also get sick far less often and avoid that all-too-common tired-out feeling that comes from my over 50-age and mostly sedentary lifestyle. Another important feature is that there are no real side effects, and no complicated programs or plans I need follow. I simply take two of each tablet several times daily and that's it. There's no confusion and most importantly - *no hassle. It's so easy, even I can do this!*

As a diabetic, I was warned to avoid artificial sugars. I was initially concerned about taking any vitamin supplement, particularly one that was fructose compounded. However, I learned through my research that one of Melaleuca's vitamins has the same amount of sugar as one cherry. I can eat one cherry and maybe even three to four cherries each day. What I shouldn't eat are several bowls of cherries. One or two? I can safely do that, live well and stay healthy.

After regularly taking Melaleuca's super-antioxidants, Cell-Wise® and vitamins, I find (and this is most clearly NOT a recommendation for anyone else to follow) I can sometimes reduce my afternoon insulin injection. I have found that sometimes my glucose counts will decrease to levels where my personal physician and primary care-giver suggests I can taper back on the amounts of insulin injected. But this is how things are with me, and in no way is this ever to be considered a recommendation for anyone else. As with all aspects pertaining to diabetes, it's important to remember: don't initiate any program separate from that approved by your regular physician or primary care-giver. Diabetes is a killer disease; plan to treat it as if your life depended upon it. It does!

Suggested Treatment: Soak feet in a tubful of warm water (or in Greg's previously mentioned ice chest). Add 1 tablespoonful Natural Spa & Bath Oil™ and 1 capful Sol-U-Mel™. After soaking for 10 to 15 minutes, dry and liberally apply T36-C7™ to any sores or lesions. As this is drying, apply a thin coating of Body Satin™ Lotion, Problem Skin Lotion™, Mela-Gel™ or even Hand Creme™. Taking some time to soak your feet will also give you an opportunity to conduct your requisite daily foot inspections.

DIAPER RASH

A common skin irritation affecting babies who have otherwise healthy skin. Friction from rough or prolonged wet diapers may contribute to the rash. Babies will vary in their susceptibility to developing diaper rash. Keeping the skin as dry as possible is one of the best methods of prevention. Diaper rash can also affect adults who are incontinent and must wear diapers.

Suggested Treatment: For diaper rashes: Add one-half ounce Sol-U-Mel™ to bath water and clean distressed area thoroughly with Anti-Bacterial Liquid Soap™. Dry thoroughly and apply Mela-Gel™ followed by either Problem Skin Lotion™ or Body Satin™ Lotion. Be sure to wash cloth diapers and clothes with MelaPower™. Add 1 capful Sol-U-Mel™ and 1 to 2 teaspoonfuls Diamond Brite™ to insure that both colors and whites will be bright and clean smelling.

EAR ACHES

Always use extreme care when treating an ear ache. When using any product, always err on the safe side of caution.

Suggested Treatment: Sharon suggests using a 100% cotton plug. She combines 1 drop T36-C7™ to 8 drops olive oil and dips the cotton in the mixture. Sharon offers this warning: Gently place the treated plug into the ear without pushing it into the ear canal. She claims this works best when the plug is left in overnight. Her *recipe* equals a 10% solution and may be appropriate for most adults. For children, she suggests a much weaker mixture, of perhaps 2-3% Melaleuca oil, or less. T36-C7™ in it's undiluted form may cause irritation to sensitive tissues. If for no other reason than this, I would always use the oil only in a very diluted form on sensitive tissue areas.

EAR (OUTER) INFECTION

Often caused by bacteria or fungus. Outer ear infections primarily afflict young adults, teenagers and are a common complaint among swimmers. Bacteria, present in rivers, lakes, pool water and the ocean, often affects the outer ear canal. Some researchers believe that an increased risk of developing ear infections may be related to long-term use of antibiotics or birth control pills.

Suggested Treatment: Dab several drops T36-C7™ on a cotton swab and apply to the outer ear twice daily. **NEVER drip pure oil into the ear canal.** This cotton swab can also be used in the same manner as the cotton ear plug under Ear Aches.

ECZEMA

An inflammation of the skin where a known cause may not be readily apparent. It may be attributed to sensitivity, toxicity or an allergy. Eczema is characterized by an outbreak of papules that frequently cause considerable itching.

Suggested Treatment: Richard, our neighbor down the road, recommends that those with eczema use **only** Problem Skin Lotion™. He suggests that those suffering from any form of eczema avoid using pure Melaleuca oil. Not all products work in the same manner for people suffering from the same condition. I have never experienced eczema, so I cannot speak from first-hand knowledge. But for those with the condition, pure Melaleuca oil does not appear to provide long-term healing.

EMPHYSEMA

A disease in which the lungs have become damaged by inhaling smoke. It is generally attributed to cigarettes either directly by smoking, or indirectly by inhaling the second-hand smoke from others. Emphysema is incurable. Damaged lung tissues do not regrow and cannot be replaced. The only effective treatment is to stop smoking, or to stop being around those who still insist on smoking.

Suggested Treatment: Many advocate inhaling pure Melaleuca alternifolia oil. Add 8 to 10 drops T36-C7™ to a vaporizer, steamer or humidifier and breathe in the warm and moist healing air. Further treatment suggestions include rubbing the chest with T36-C7™ followed by Pain-A-Trate™. The outlook for those suffering from emphysema is not good, particularly if there has been extensive lung damage. Eventually, emphysema will cause heart failure or respiratory collapse. Now, is this sufficient reason to stop smoking?

FEVER BLISTER

See Cold Sores.

FUNGAL INFECTION OUTBREAKS

Diseases principally of the skin, but which can affect other organs. Outbreaks can range from mild and unnoticed to severe and even fatal. Fungal infections are common and more serious in those who take long-term antibiotics or who have immune deficiency disorders such as AIDS. They are opportunistic infections since they take advantage of a victim's lowered defenses.

Fungal infections are commonly found in those with diabetes. Warm moist areas, such as in skin folds or between the toes, encourage the development of fungal skin infections. The majority of such infections are superficial and include thrush, jock itch, ringworm, nail infection and athlete's foot. Deep infections, while uncommon, are more frequent particularly in those having compromised immune systems.

Suggested Treatment: For common fungal infections, wash the affected areas with Anti-Bacterial Liquid Soap™. Dry and apply Problem Skin Lotion™ or Body Satin™ Lotion. For acute outbreaks apply T36-C7™ followed by Mela-Gel™ or Triple Antibiotic Ointment™. Repeat regularly at least 2 to 3 times daily for 7 to 10 days. If no improvement is noted, or if the condition deteriorates, contact your physician or primary care-giver.

FURUNCLE

See Boils.

GANGRENE

A medical term for the death of tissue resulting from loss of or diminished blood supply caused by the narrowing of arteries and vessels. While it can affect any area of the body, gangrene generally appears on the feet, legs, fingers and arms. The majority of the estimated 50,000 non-traumatic amputations annually in America are performed on diabetics.

Other causes for gangrene include arteriosclerosis, thrombosis, embolism and frostbite. Amputation is not always required, particularly if aggressive treatment can be initiated immediately. In an earlier chapter, results from a 1936 study mentioned Melaleuca alternifolia oil's effectiveness in treating and reversing diabetic gangrene.

Suggested Treatment: There are reports of people with sores that could have led to gangrene, who were able to heal their sores with frequent applications of T36-C7™ and T40-C5™. For them it worked! *Now that I know about the benefits of Melaleuca alternifolia oil, I intend to keep my toes and feet in as good a condition as possible. I always keep a good supply of both T36-C7™ and T40-C5™ with me.*

HOWEVER, if any deterioration in the feet and toes is noted, the diabetic should ***immediately*** contact their physician or primary care-giver.

GINGIVITIS

Periodontal or gum disease that is due to infection in the gum tissues. It is usually caused by a build-up of plaque. Some believe that toxins within the plaque irritate the gums and cause gingivitis. It often results in infection and swollen gums that bleed easily during or after even gentle-to-moderate brushing and flossing.

I overheard my young nephew Bradley explaining gingivitis to one of his contemporaries, telling her that this was something that older people get when they eat too many ginger snaps and drink too much coffee.

Suggested Treatment: Brush teeth daily with Melaleuca's Tooth Polish and floss with Dental Tape™. If condition is severe, apply T36-C7™ to your finger or a cotton swab and dab it on the affected gum areas. Rinsing with Breath-Away™ Mouth Wash and using Hot Shot™ Mouth & Throat Spray may also help alleviate gingivitis.

GUM DISEASE

Periodontal disease should be a concern to everyone. Conditions range from a mild inflammation to severe gum recession and caries. Inflammation of the gums, or gingivitis, is the most common gum disease and is due primarily to infection within the tissues.

Suggested Treatment: Use a cotton swab or your finger to apply T36-

C7™ directly on the affected region. Use Melaleuca's Tooth Polish and Breath-Away™ Mouth Wash several times daily. T36-C7™ soothes inflamed gum tissues and, *while it does not have one of the greatest tastes in the world, it does taste like it is working and accelerating the healing process.*

HALITOSIS

Common ailment that affects millions. It is often caused by a microbial overgrowth in the mouth. Sometimes it is indicative of an internal dysfunction. If halitosis cannot be readily relieved, then secondary causes should be investigated with your physician or primary care-giver.

Suggested Treatment: Frequently use Melaleuca's Tooth Polish and Breath-Away™ Mouth Wash. Sometimes halitosis, or bad breath, is caused by intestinal parasites, constipation or some untreated serious disease such as cancer. As stated frequently throughout these pages, if any treatment idea suggested doesn't work as well as you think it should, by all means consult your physician or primary care-giver.

HEAD LICE

Causes pain, itching and irritation, head lice feed off blood obtained when they bite. Lice generally affect the scalp but also can attack other areas including extremities and genitals. Infestations occur where there is shared contact with items such as hats or combs and brushes. Outbreaks are common in schools and close-living situations. While infestations are generally localized, they can involve such tiny areas as the eyebrows and eyelashes where they latch onto hair strands. A magnifying glass is often needed to see the small grayish-white ova typical of head lice.

Suggested Treatment: Pour a quantity of T36-C7™ on your hands or scalp and massage-in thoroughly before combing through the hair. Then, wrap the head with a hot moist towel. Make certain that your "hot" is not "burning hot". Don't compound the lice problem with a head scalding problem. Keep the towel in place for 8 to 10 minutes before shampooing. Use Natural Shampoo™ or Melaleuca's Herbal Shampoo™ and wash hair at least twice daily for 7 to 10 days. Repeat this entire process (including massaging in the oil and wrapping the head with a hot moist towel) in two days. Do this even if you don't notice any additional head lice.

To avoid lice re-infestation wash all clothes, towels and bedding that have been in contact with the infected person. Use 1/8th cupful MelaPower™ and 1 to 2 capfuls Sol-U-Mel™ per wash load.

HEADACHE

Any head pain, ranging from a dull throbbing throughout the head, to a sharp, searing or localized pain. An estimated 35,000,000 Americans endure chronic headaches. 18,000,000 suffer from headache pain so severe it will disrupt their every-day life. Probably the most severe type of headache is the migraine, an intense throbbing pain that is usually located on either side of the head. Other types of headaches include those associated with caffeine withdrawal. These headaches can last several days or until the next jolt of caffeine from coffee, chocolate, over-the-counter drugs, tea or soda pop. Sinus headaches generally cause pain across the cheeks, forehead, nose and behind the eyes. Tension headaches, the most common, can cause pain all over the head and the back of the neck.

Suggested Treatment: Many obtain headache pain relief by using T36-C7™ followed by Pain-A-Trate™. Be careful so you don't drip either Melaleuca product on sensitive tissue areas near your eyes or ears.

HEMORRHOIDS

Characterized by enlarged varicose veins in the anus wall. There is considerable argument about the cause. Hemorrhoids can be brought on by pregnancy, lack of dietary fiber, diarrhea, constipation or activities that require sitting for extended periods on hard or cold surfaces. When external hemorrhoids strangulate, they can develop gangrene. Preventing gangrene may require alternative treatments from your physician or primary caregiver. If your hemorrhoid condition is severe, do not hesitate to seek professional treatment and advice.

Suggested Treatment: Combine 1 teaspoonful Sol-U-Mel™ and 1 capful Natural Spa & Bath Oil™ with 1 cup lukewarm water. Stir to combine well. Gently sponge the solution onto the hemorrhoidal area. Leave on for several minutes before carefully drying. Apply T36-C7™; then follow with Problem Skin Lotion™. Continue treatment for 7 to 10 days. Steve suggests he obtains extra relief by soaking in a hot bath with 1 capful Sol-U-Mel™ and 1 capful Spa & Bath Oil™ added to the water.

Please note that as with every other treatment suggestion or idea presented in these pages, if there is no improvement noted within a reasonable time, contact your physician or primary care-giver.

HEMORRHOIDS - BLEEDING

Ted suggests combining 1 to 2 capfuls Nature's Cleanse™ in an enema bottle filled with warm (definitely not hot!) water, and using as an enema. He asserts that this has helped him stop his hemorrhoidal bleeding for as long as 1 week. However, I think it's really important to add a precautionary warning statement: **If you have rectal bleeding, contact your physician or primary care-giver** (to determine the exact cause or nature of such bleeding) ***before*** improvising any type of alternative treatment, including this one.

INGROWN TOE NAIL

A painful condition that usually affects the big toe. The nail presses into the adjacent skin area and causes inflammation and infection. There is a difference of opinion as to what causes ingrown toe nails. Florence believes it is caused by poor personal hygiene. Brett claims it's caused by improperly trimming toe nails. Others attribute ingrown nails to wearing shoes that are too small.

To trim toe nails properly, doctors suggest reshaping the nail with a "v" in the middle. This allows the nail to draw in towards the center and prevents the edges from piercing the skin. Others suggest cutting the nails straight across. They believe rounded trimming should be avoided. *With all this divergent opinion out there in the countryside, there must be a lot of people suffering from ingrown toe nails. Fortunately I am not one of them.*

Suggested Treatment: Soak the affected foot for 20 minutes in a solution of 1 capful Sol-U-Mel™ added to 16 ounces water. Dry and apply T36-C7™ followed by Problem Skin Lotion™ or Mela-Gel™. Repeat this procedure in the morning and again before bedtime. Continue treatment until the inflamed area has healed and the nail can be properly trimmed.

INSECT BITES & STINGS

Should be treated the same as any injury or wound. They often have the potential for developing infection. The world contains nearly 1,000,000 known species of insects. Most are harmless to humans and many are beneficial. Flies and insects that bite are the most troublesome.

Suggested Treatment: *Those allergic to insect bites and stings should follow the instructions in their antidote kit.* Apply T36-C7™ to the bite area. This will stop the pain and itching almost immediately. Follow with applications of Mela-Gel™, Triple Antibiotic Ointment™ or Problem Skin Lotion™. In situations where there are numerous bites, or where the bites are more serious, prepare a hot pack using 1 tablespoonful Sol-U-Mel™ and 1 capful Natural Spa & Bath Oil™ combined in a cupful of warm water. Dampen a cloth with this mixture and place on the bite areas. Repeat as necessary.

INSOMNIA

Affects an estimated one-third of all American adults at one time or another. Probably the most common cause of sleeplessness is worry. Insomnia can be caused by a physical problem, too much caffeine (that extra cup of coffee stretching past 8 p.m.), too little daytime exercise, anxiety or depression, or withdrawal from cigarettes, drugs, liquor or addictive substances.

Suggested Treatment: For common insomnia, I will recommend a treatment that usually works for me: I try to calm my mind, slow the thought process down and take a break from myself. If this doesn't work, I will fix a cup or two of G'Day™ Melaleuca Tea and acknowledge that it has been a good day. I can then sit back, relax and know that tomorrow will hold other challenges and new goals. *Actually, this is a great idea! I'll change my coffee pot over to brewing a potful of G'Day™ Melaleuca Tea and then try to finish this chapter by breakfast. You see, I'm writing this at 3:30 a.m., because I couldn't sleep - either.*

ITCHY & FLAKY SKIN

May indicate other problems such as allergies, psoriasis or perhaps a nutritional deficiency.

Suggested Treatment: Regularly take vitamins from The Vitality Pak™. Wash daily with Anti-Bacterial Liquid Soap™ or the Gold Bar™. Apply Problem Skin Lotion™, Body Satin™ Lotion or Hand Creme™. Nancy suggests using either Sun-Shades 9™ or Sun-Shades 15™ since both are very moisturizing. Whichever Melaleuca oil/lotion you use, continue treatments at least twice daily for 10 to 14 days.

JOCK ITCH

A common fungal infection found in the moist skin fold areas of the body. Fungi and yeasts such as candida, thrive in moist environments and are responsible for jock itch. Often this condition forms lesions around one or both sides of the crotch area. Since scratching or rubbing enhances the fungi and makes symptoms worse, it should be avoided. While jock itch generally occurs in warm weather, in the summer or in times and places where humidity is high, the condition is chronic. This means that the fungi will continue to re-infect, time and again, those most susceptible to developing it.

Suggested Treatment: Wash the affected area with Anti-Bacterial Liquid Soap™. Pat dry and lightly apply T36-C7™. Follow with Problem Skin Lotion™. Repeat twice daily. Bob advocates applying T40-C5™ followed by ordinary corn starch, claiming that keeping the area dry (after allowing the Melaleuca oil to absorb into the area) is his main concern. However, if neither suggestion works for you, consult your physician or primary care-giver.

Melaleuca alternifolia oil is more effective than other treatment options, particularly when considering the rapidity of results following application, relief of symptoms, high cure ratios and cost effectiveness. Many reduce their chances for re-infection by cleaning bathroom areas using a 16 ounce spray bottle containing 2 capfuls Tough 'N Tender™, 10 drops T36-C7™ and 2 capfuls Sol-U-Mel™. When sprayed on and wiped off, this sanitizes the bathroom and helps eliminate further fungal outbreaks.

LYME DISEASE

Characterized by skin changes, joint inflammation and flu-like symptoms including fever, headache, lethargy and muscle pains. It is transmitted by a tick that usually lives on deer, but can sometimes live on dogs.

Treatment Suggestions: See Arthritis and/or Insect Bite Suggestions.

Preventative Suggestions: Applying liberal amounts of T36-C7™, Sun-Screen 9™ or 15™, Body Satin™ Lotion, Hand Creme™ or Orchard Mist™ Hair Spray before walking in the woods appears to inhibit ticks and insect bites.

MIGRAINE HEADACHES

Best described as having severe headache pain that can last from a few hours to several days. Migraines are frequently accompanied by vision problems, nausea and vomiting. Causes for migraines are unknown. Some suspected causes are: heredity, stress or depression, diabetes, seasonal changes, bright lights, loud music, birth control pills or indulging in foods such as chocolate, dairy products or wine.

Suggested Treatment: Many who suffer from migraines obtain significant relief after applying Pain-A-Trate™ on their temples, forehead and the back of their neck. Be careful that the oil does not drip on eyelids or other sensitive skin areas. Pain-A-Trate™ penetrates the skin and works deep in tissues as it helps relieve severe pain.

MOSQUITO BITES

If you have ever endured a summer in the Upper Midwest without mosquitoes, it must have been the one when snow was still around in July and August. Minnesota is known for two seasons - Winter and Mosquitoes. I never leave home in the summer without taking my Melaleuca alternifolia oil with me. It repels even Minnesota mosquitoes.

Suggested Treatment: Jenny applies T36-C7™ to her bites and follows with Problem Skin Lotion™ or Body Satin™ Lotion. Applying Melaleuca's products just before going outside into a mosquito infested environment (which in Minnesota can mean nearly everywhere) really helps keep the little critters away. *Products I use for my preventative program include Orchard Mist™ Hair Spray* (applied to the strands I have left) *and the various lotions mentioned in these pages.* Be sure to read Russ' recipe for mosquito control under the "Chore List With Suggested Remedies" chapter.

MOUTH ULCERS

See Canker Sores.

Muscle Aches

Often the result of over-exertion, sports, exercise and going through too many turns and twists in the motions of everyday living.

Just the thought of yard work makes my old muscles ache. So does trying to do more than I should at my age. Come to think of it, even when I was younger, my muscles would stage revolts and often ache. Maybe that's another trick of memory: perhaps it was me staging the revolt against doing all the yard work, rather than the fault of the yard work itself.

I've found that Access™ bars help prevent and eliminate cramps, sore muscles, a sore back and that all around ache that says I've pushed too hard that day. As a diabetic, I've discovered that before commencing any sustained exercise or activity, by eating just one-third of an Access™ bar, most of the body parts that once (prior to my being introduced to this amazing bar) ached and became sore - simply don't. Another benefit is that I have more energy and am then better equipped to accomplish the very activity that once caused my muscles to ache. All this, without creating any new aches or pains. I would urge all diabetics to first talk with their physician or primary caregiver before trying the Access™ bars. In my initial "experiments", I checked my glucose levels before consuming part of a bar and then rechecked the levels frequently during my exercise or work periods. This allowed me to determine exactly how the Access™ bar worked for me as I developed my own quantity-and-use schedule.

I suppose all this talk about diabetics and diabetes is boring to readers who are neither and don't know any diabetics. I could offer a smart answer, but I'll avoid that at the suggestion of my weary editors and offer the next paragraph instead.

Non-diabetics can often consume up to a whole bar within 20 minutes or so before commencing any planned exercise or similar type of activity. There are many stories from runners and joggers, lifters and physical workout specialists, and even from the more ordinary others who exercise, relating the value of Access™ bars. They claim it improves their ability to accomplish more without muscle aches and pains. However, for those who still suffer from muscle aches, the following suggestion may help alleviate the condition.

Suggested Treatment: I have had excellent results when I liberally apply Pain-A-Trate™. Sometimes I follow with Body Satin™ Lotion. Mary recommends applying T36-C7™ first, followed by Pain-A-Trate™. She believes this enhances the action of the Pain-A-Trate™ and allows the oil to reach down deep to soothe aching muscles.

As an addendum, just mentioning the word "effects" makes me mindful of telling you that I particularly enjoy the "before-effects" and the "after-effects" of an evening spent applying Body Satin™ Lotion to a favorite body.... Talk about relieving an aching muscle or two. Even at my age, I can add a definite -wow!

Avoid dripping the pure oil on or around the eyes, eyelids or other sensitive tissue areas. Melaleuca oil is an effective penetrating oil, so be careful when using it.

NASAL CONGESTION

Partial blockage of a nasal passage caused by an inflammation of the mucous membrane. Congestion can be the result of an infection of the passageway resulting from a cold, an infection coming from the sinuses, or allergies.

Suggested Treatment: Add 5 to 10 drops T36-C7™ to a steam vaporizer and breathe in the healthy moist air. Sometimes when I am particularly congested, I will also apply T36-C7™ to my forehead, cheeks, the bridge of my nose, and directly under my nose.

OBESITY

25% of all Americans are overweight and carry too much body fat for their bone structure. *My doctor tells me that obesity occurs when the net energy intake exceeds the net energy expenditure. I asked him, "Does this mean I should eat less?" He replied, "Yes, and move around more, too." Now, I understand!*

Another way to say this, is that obesity results when more calories are consumed than are used by the body. Individual energy requirements are based in part on a person's metabolism, and part on their activity level. While genetics may play a part, a sedentary life style contributes.

Obesity increases the chances of becoming seriously ill. High blood pressure, stroke, coronary heart disease and other conditions are more common in an obese person than in someone who is lean. Diabetes is five times more likely in those who are obese. Women who are overweight show a corresponding increase in the risk of developing breast, uterine and cervical cancer. Osteoarthritis is aggravated by obesity. Obese men have a greater risk of developing cancer of the colon, rectum and prostate.

Okay, so those are the facts. Those among us, including this writer, are aware of all of this. So, what can we do? Diets do not work by themselves. As someone who is getting older, jumping up and down in a wild aerobics exercise seems okay when watching Jane Fonda. But let's face it, I will never look like the men she jumps with. So, what's my alternative to finally and forever rid this larger-than-should-be body from all this extra weight?

How about Melaleuca's Access™ bar? Yes. It works. Friends, there is help for us obese souls who do not like the jumping up and down exercises. I can peddle my $5 exercise bike (bought at my local Salvation Army store) and I can still walk. Plus, after consuming even part of an Access™ bar, I know that some of my fat will start to burn off. *You know, this is easy even for me. Best of all, it is fairly fast. I am losing weight and getting healthier. Now, how about you?*

You have all the reasons and there are no more excuses. No one will get healthy for you. There is no proxy possible here!

As a diabetic I tried just 1/3 of an Access™ bar. I waited 20 minutes and tested my glucose. When it did not climb higher, I started my daily walk confident that I was then starting to burn off fat from my first step. Of course I always carry my diabetic kit with me and bring along some hard candy and several sugar packets in the event I start feeling weak or shaky. Access™ bars are working for me and while I have not had to have my pants taken in yet, I am hopeful that will come next. If you are diabetic, or know someone who is, introduce them to the Access™ bar and Melaleuca's other life-saving, life-enhancing products. I absolutely know they will be extremely grateful.

OSTEOARTHRITIS

See Arthritis.

PARONYCHIA

An infection of the tissue around a toe nail or finger nail that is caused by yeast or bacteria. The infection may follow a nail and extend underneath it to where it can penetrate deeply into tendons and muscle tissue. Eventually, if not treated properly, the infection may distort the nail and interfere with its normal function.

Suggested Treatment: Wash well using Anti-Bacterial Liquid Soap™. Soak the affected nail for 10 to 15 minutes in a quart of warm water to which you have added 1 capful Natural Spa & Bath Oil™ and 1 capful Sol-U-Mel™. Dry well and apply T40-C5™ on the affected nail.

PIMPLES

See Acne.

POISON IVY

Contains a powerful irritating oil that causes a distinct line-like rash wherever contact has been made with the skin. Poison Ivy appears as a plant, bush or vine and has three shiny leaves on each stem. The leaves turn red in the fall. In late summer, it has white flowers or cream-colored berries. Even in winter when the leaves have dropped, the plant can still be quite toxic.

Suggested Treatment: To relieve the pain and itching, clean affected area with Anti-Bacterial Liquid Soap™. Pat dry and apply T36-C7™ followed by Problem Skin Lotion™ or Mela-Gel™.

POISON OAK

Contains a powerful irritating oil that causes a distinct line-like rash wherever it makes contact with the skin. It is commonly found in sandy soil and pine woods along both the West and East Coasts. Poison Oak has shiny green oak-like leaves clustered in groups of 3 or 5.

Suggested Treatment: Follow the same suggestions as recommended for Poison Ivy.

POISON SUMAC

Has the same characteristics of the two preceding plants. It is a short shrub or small tree having smooth gray bark and branches with 7 to 13 dull green leaflets. The leaves turn yellow in autumn. White berries distinguish it from the harmless sumacs. The poison variety predominantly grows in swampy areas or along streams.

Special Treatment Note: If you come in contact with Poison Ivy, Poison Oak or Poison Sumac, wash whatever has been contaminated. For clothing, use 1/8th cupful MelaPower™ and 2 capfuls Sol-U-Mel™ per wash load. For tools or steering wheels or anything mechanical, mix 1 part each of Tough 'N Tender™ and Sol-U-Mel™ to 5 parts water. Spray on and allow it to stand for several minutes before wiping dry. Do not try to destroy these plants by burying or burning leaves or root systems. Burying will spread the plant. Burning will expose the skin, eyes, nose and throat to greater harm from inhaling smoke.

PSORIASIS

A chronic skin disease characterized by itchy, dry and thick scaly red patches. This usually appears on forearms, elbows, knees, legs, scalp, armpits, groin, eyebrows, under the nails and even in the ears. Patches can vary from several lesions to a widespread attack that can also include disabling arthritis. Generally, psoriasis lesions heal without scarring.

Suggested Treatment: Use Anti-Bacterial Liquid Soap™ or the Gold Bar™. For a relaxing soak, fill a tub with warm water and add 1 to 2 capfuls Natural Spa & Bath Oil™. After drying, apply T36-C7™ followed by Problem Skin Lotion™ or Mela-Gel™. Repeat twice daily. Some claim using Body Satin™ Lotion will control outbreaks. If the outbreak is under the nail, apply T40-C5™. For further treatment suggestions, see "Paronychia". Consult your physician or primary care-giver if the condition does not improve within a reasonable time.

PRURITIS

Clinical name for "itchy skin". This condition may indicate something more serious. It could be a sign of allergies, internal fungal infection, cancer, hepatitis, kidney problems or potential liver failure. Now after that scare, I will tell you that it could also be the result of a vitamin deficiency, dry skin, or allergic reaction to something in your life that can easily be changed or altered.

Suggested Treatment: In most instances, itching can be alleviated by bathing with Anti-Bacterial Liquid Soap™ or the Gold Bar™. Apply Problem Skin Lotion™ or Body Satin™ Lotion. If an itchy area has been scratched and the skin surface broken, first treat with T36-C7™. If the condition continues for longer than 7 to 10 days, see your physician or primary care-giver.

PUNCTURE WOUNDS

Stabbing wounds that break the skin's surface. When punctured, the immediate area becomes red and inflamed. White blood cells that fight infection rush to the wound. As puncture wounds heal, scabs form a natural bandage that protects the wound.

Suggested Treatment: Cleanse with Anti-Bacterial Liquid Soap™. Pat dry and apply T36-C7™. Follow with Problem Skin Lotion™ Mela-Gel™ or Triple Antibiotic Ointment™. Puncture wounds heal faster and have less opportunity to develop infections if you use this treatment as soon as an injury occurs. If you are somewhere where you cannot easily clean the wound, apply T36-C7™. Melaleuca alternifolia oil penetrates deeply into injured tissues and delivers healing to distressed sites. A wound can always be washed later.

Note: Tetanus can occur when wounds are deep or contaminated. If it has been more than 5 years since you have had a tetanus shot, immediately contact your physician or primary care-giver. The majority of victims dying from tetanus are older adults who have not kept current on booster shots.

RASHES

An eruption on the skin characterized by redness and welts.

Suggested Treatment: I have effectively treated several unknown-origin rashes by using this mixture: 1 capful Natural Spa & Bath Oil™ added to 1 cupful water. Dab this solution on the rash. Pat dry and apply Problem Skin Lotion™ or Mela-Gel™. T36-C7™ is also effective when treating rashes.

RED EYE (STYES)

A pus-filled sore or abscess often found near the inside corner of the eye or along the eye lid. Styes can often be very painful.

Suggested Treatment: Many people find relief when placing a damp tea bag over the closed lid of the affected eye. *That's right folks - use a G'Day™ Melaleuca Tea bag! I am told that it really works!*

Ringworm

Commonly appears in the crotch, feet, scalp and trunk portions of the body. The fungi that causes it grows in moist areas. For treatment suggestions, refer to "Jock Itch" and "Athlete's Foot".

Suggested Treatment: Wash the affected area with Anti-Bacterial Liquid Soap™. Pat dry and lightly apply T36-C7™, followed by Problem Skin Lotion™. Repeat this process at least twice daily until the condition has cleared.

Rough Skin on Elbows/Knees/Heels

When showering use the Gold Bar™ on all rough skin areas. Alternate between Anti-Bacterial Liquid Soap™ and the Gold Bar™. After drying, apply Body Satin™ Lotion or Hand Creme™. Some prefer using Problem Skin Lotion™. Most of my problems with rough skin have been on my heels and feet. *I have discovered that it doesn't seem to matter which Melaleuca lotion I use since each produces good results. Generally, problem areas have cleared after several applications. These days I use either Body Satin™ Lotion or Hand Creme™. I haven't experienced rough skin since switching to products containing Melaleuca alternifolia oil.*

Scabies

Caused by an easily transmittable "itch-mite" or parasitic infection. They cause intense itching. Often they seem to prefer webs and secret places such as around a woman's nipple area and on a male's genitals. Scabies, or crabs, can even appear in finger webs, arm pits, along the belt line and sometimes the lower buttocks. Proper diagnosis is confirmed through microscopic inspection.

Suggested Treatment: Fill a tub with hot water and add 2 capfuls Natural Spa & Bath Oil™ and 1 capful Sol-U-Mel™. Soak for 20 minutes. Dry and apply T36-C7™ followed by Problem Skin Lotion™ or Body Satin™ Lotion. Repeat twice daily. Wash all clothes, towels and bedding using 1/8th cupful MelaPower™. Add at least 2 capfuls Sol-U-Mel™ and 1 to 2 teaspoonfuls Diamond Brite™ to each load.

Seborrhea

Primarily affects adults. It appears around the scalp, face and other body areas usually as a dry or greasy scaling. Sometimes seborrhea is confused with thick dandruff. In severe cases it may appear as a yellow or red scaling along the hairline and behind the ears, external ear canals, eyebrows and nasal folds. Seborrhea is more prevalent in winter months. Climate conditions and genetic predisposition can affect the severity.

Suggested Treatment: Bathe affected areas with Anti-Bacterial Liquid Soap™ or the Gold Bar™. Dry and apply T36-C7™ followed by Problem Skin Lotion™ or Mela-Gel™. Continue twice daily. Body Satin™ Lotion and regular use of Natural Shampoo™ is also effective.

SHINGLES

Caused by the same virus as chicken pox. Shingles generally affect adults. Rather than repeating the Chicken Pox treatment suggestions, jump back a few pages and read my words.

SINUS CONGESTION

Caused by a minor infection, a reaction to an environmental cause or an allergy. Often it can be attributed to cigarette or cigar smoke, dust, chemicals, pollen or any of the hundreds of other airborne particles that launch effective attacks against us. Melaleuca alternifolia oil is excellent in opening blocked respiratory passages and killing bacteria and microbes. It also will alleviate sinus congestion and clear lung ailments including cough, pneumonia and influenza.

Suggested Treatment: Dab a few drops T36-C7™ directly under the nose and sinus areas. Mela-Gel™ also provides significant relief when dabbed under the nose. Add 1 to 2 capfuls Sol-U-Mel™ and 10 drops T36-C7™ to a vaporizer. Rub T36-C7™ followed by Pain-A-Trate™ liberally on the upper chest. *Either treatment method works for me. Maybe that's because I tend to "throw a lot" of Melaleuca at whatever ailment I develop.*

SINUSITIS

An inflammation of the mucous lined air spaces often caused by an infection spreading from the nose.

Suggested Treatment: Follow the directions under Sinus Congestion, above.

SORE GUMS

Have you ever experienced the ache and agony of sore gums? Until Melaleuca, it was just another chronic ache and pain I thought I would have to endure without complaint. I was wrong; I can complain. Only trouble is - now I don't have *that* to complain about anymore.

Suggested Treatment: My sore gums healed when I applied T36-C7™. I also switched to Melaleuca's Tooth Polish. If you're experiencing sore gums, perhaps there is another reason for your condition. Maybe you have something as simple as a mineral deficiency that can be alleviated by switching to Mel-Vita™ and Mela-Cal™ multi-vitamin and multi-mineral supplements.

However, sore gums can also be caused by tooth problems. When was your last checkup? *You know, these days with Melaleuca oil, one shouldn't have to endure "a sore anything" for very long.*

SORE THROATS

Are often the body's first indication of an oncoming cold or flu. In children, a sore throat can precede chicken pox, mumps, colds and measles. If a sore throat continues for longer than several days, your physician or primary care-giver should be consulted.

Suggested Treatment: Plan to gargle with a solution of 10 drops T36-C7™ diluted in 1/4 cup of warm water. Or try swabbing the back of your throat with a long cotton swab saturated with T36-C7™. Personally, I've tried both methods and prefer neither *(believing the gargling solution more resembles an oil slick on a spring swamp than something that actually will heal my aching throat...).*

Generally, to alleviate sore throats, I use Hot Shot™ Mouth & Throat Spray and drink copious amounts of G'Day™ Melaleuca Tea. Getting plenty of rest is important, too. In my bedside vaporizer, I add 1 capful Sol-U-Mel™ and 10 to 15 drops T36-C7™. I enjoy (really) gargling with Breath-Away™ Mouth Wash. *So far, these remedies have helped me and I have not yet had to test my manhood again by gargling with that T36-C7™ mixture.*

SPORTS INJURIES & SPRAINS

These occur in both contact and non-contact sports, as well as from all types of physical activities. Injuries are common in combative sports such as hockey and football. Other sports such as soccer, baseball and basketball also produce their share of injuries. Most injuries sustained are relatively minor and limited to cuts and bruises. More serious injuries affect ligaments, joints and soft-tissue areas.

Melaleuca alternifolia oil is now used by many professional sports people. They apply it as soon as an injury occurs, even before cleansing the wound. Melaleuca alternifolia oil is an antiseptic and anti-inflammatory agent that safeguards injured sites from secondary germ contamination. Sprains respond well to the oil because it reduces swelling while numbing pain.

Suggested Treatment: When possible, wash the area with Anti-Bacterial Liquid Soap™. Dry and liberally apply T36-C7™ followed by Pain-A-Trate™, Problem Skin Lotion™ or Body Satin™ Lotion. Repeat as often as necessary until both the swelling and pain have subsided.

STINGING NETTLES

Found in wooded areas throughout the U.S. and Canada. This perennial plant is characterized by having finely toothed heart-shaped leaves that look somewhat like those of a strawberry plant. The nettles have stems with hair-like needles that sting when they touch or brush against skin.

Suggested Treatment: Apply adhesive tape to the affected areas. As you gently lift the tape, the smaller needles will come off. Immediately apply T36-C7™ to the affected area before using a tweezer to extract the remaining larger needles. After the removal process, wash gently with Anti-Bacterial Liquid Soap™. Pat dry and apply T36-C7™ followed by Mela-Gel™ or Triple Antibiotic Ointment™. Repeat this treatment at least every 1 to 2 hours until the irritation subsides.

SUNBURN

Caused by an over-exposure to the sun that results in inflammation of the skin. When ordinary skin is sunburned, it becomes tender as it turns red. Sometimes the skin can blister. In extreme cases sunburn can cause sunstroke and collapse. Multiple mild cases can cause premature aging.

Suggested Treatment: Apply T36-C7™ to the sunburned areas, then liberally apply Sun-Shades 9™. Massage gingerly into the burned areas to avoid additional irritation. Follow with Problem Skin Lotion™ or Body Satin™ Lotion. Repeat as needed. Refer to "Burns" for additional treatment.

THRUSH (ORAL)

Can affect anyone. Oral thrush often affects people with compromised immune systems such as those suffering from HIV and AIDS. Others susceptible to thrush include those on chemotherapy or cortisone. Melaleuca alternifolia oil is an effective treatment for oral thrush. It may also sometimes be used by infants and pregnant women in a **VERY** diluted form. People with severe or life-threatening illness should consult with their physician or primary care-giver before using Melaleuca oil.

Suggested Treatment: Use a long cotton swab or finger to apply T36-C7™ to affected tissues. This will help alleviate pain and itching. Those people with sensitive mucous membranes should not use more than a 5-10% concentration of pure oil. Oral thrush outbreaks are very difficult to cure. Repeated applications will be needed to effectively eradicate lesions.

TICKS

Ticks are small, 8-legged bugs that attach themselves to human (or animal) skin where they feed on the blood. Ticks may be picked up when walking in (generally) rural or suburban yards and woods, in long grass and scrub lands. They can also be brought home by dogs running free. Some ticks may attach themselves and go unnoticed for several hours; others can cause pain, bruising and even severe irritation. Some ticks carry Lyme Disease, others carry Rocky Mountain Spotted Fever; certain ticks also are known to be carriers of viral encephalitis. Some ticks can be extremely harmful, particularly to the very young or the very old; in rare instances, they emit a dangerous toxin that can ultimately result in paralysis and death.

Suggested Treatment: Combine a few drops T36-C7™ with 1 part Sol-U-Mel™ and 3 parts water. Apply 3 to 5 drops to the tick. Don't try to pull the tick off from wherever it has attached itself. Most often, the stinger will remain in the skin and cause subsequent infection. If the tick doesn't immediately die from the solution you have "tickled" it with, use several drops of T36-C7™. After you've removed the tick, clean the site with Anti-Bacterial Liquid Soap™. Then dry thoroughly and apply T36-C7™ and Mela-Gel™; repeat these applications at least several times per hour, or as often as necessary. If fever or any other conditions develop, contact your physician or primary care-giver.

WARTS

A hard benign growth caused by a virus. They can occur anywhere on the body: hands, fingers, legs and knees, elbows and sometimes the face. Melaleuca alternifolia oil can often eliminate warts within several weeks of initiating a consistent schedule of applications.

Suggested Treatment: Apply T40-C5™ morning and evening. Soak the wart area (if possible) in a solution of 1 capful Natural Spa & Bath Oil™ and 1 capful Sol-U-Mel™ in a gallon of warm water. Or, rinse a cloth in this solution and cover the wart. Keep in place for 10 minutes.

WASP STINGS

Usually stings are immediately painful causing an immediate surprise type of pain. The site that has been stung usually will become red and sore.

NOTE: If you're allergic to wasp stings, follow the directions in your antidote kit. Immediately seek proper medical assistance; your life can depend on the action you take, and the action taken by others around you. **Wasp stings can be life-threatening. Act as if your life depended upon obtaining treatment.**

Other Suggested Treatment: Medical experts recommend that you first inspect the bite area to determine if the stinger is still in the skin. If possible, remove it (carefully) without squeezing; your goal is to avoid breaking the venom sack. Nancy and Andy sell honey in New England; they claim they've discovered excellent sting relief when applying T36-C7™ followed by Mela-Gel™, every 15 minutes for 6 to 8 applications. We mention bee stings in a wasp suggestion because according to those who best know, most stings are pretty much the same when it comes to comparing pain and when offering treatment suggestions.

*Other than my previously mentioned walk in a strawberry patch and the result-ing sting, I've cautiously avoided nearly all contact with wasps and bees. I've grown to respect them and whatever reasonable territory they want to use. If they stake a claim on a particular area, I can respect that and go work in another part of the yard. Or I can use my Sol-U-Mel™ loaded spray if the respect is not mutual and if we cannot arrive at a reasonably harmonious relationship in **my** gardens.*

YEAST INFECTIONS

A generalized term that includes a variety of problems including vaginal infection, inflammation and irritation. Infections can be caused by parasites, viruses, fungi or bacteria. Inflammation and irritation may be attributable to chemicals in tampons, bubble baths and tissue paper. Sometimes excessive use of harsh soap will cause vaginitis.

Clothing contributes to yeast infections, particularly in those containing synthetic fibers such as polyester and nylon. Synthetic clothing retains mois-ture and encourages yeast growth. Bacteria can remain in synthetic fibers even after washing.

Those familiar with Melaleuca's products, know that washing clothes in MelaPower™ and adding 1 capful of Sol-U-Mel™ to each wash load will leave clothes organism-free, safe and clean.

Incidents of yeast infection are more common today than they were three decades ago. Excessive or prolonged use of antibiotics destroys normal bac-teria flora. This over-growth of fungus and yeast causes vaginitis.

Yeast infections are a common complaint of women. Symptoms include pain, itching, spotting, odor, irritation and discharge. Recurrent or chronic infections will develop frequently in those who are diabetic, and in those tak-ing birth control pills or antibiotics. Symptoms can be alleviated for many, however the majority will not be cured by traditional treatments.

Suggested Treatment: Use Nature's Cleanse™ according to package direc-tions. **Melaleuca alternifolia oil is the only antiseptic capable of elimi-nating each of the major types of vaginal yeast infections while exhibit-ing virtually no toxicity to vaginal tissues.** *Clearly, Melaleuca alternifolia oil and Nature's Cleanse™ are "near-miracle products".*

ADDENDUM

This listing of conditions that respond to Melaleuca alternifolia oil or products containing the oil, is still incomplete. But, a good rule-of-thumb is the one we use at our house: General preventative care means that everyone here routinely takes Melaleuca's vitamins. We're all adults and mostly con-firmed coffee drinkers. Yet, we've learned to drink at least several potfuls of G'Day™ Melaleuca Tea each day. Have you tried this tea ice-cold? I think it's about the best year-round drink available; it tastes just as good iced in the winter months as it does in the few months we call summer. Plus, it's far better for your health and far cheaper than drinking soda pop. Our after-minor-injury-care means we always reach for a Melaleuca medicine chest product first. In all our combined years, we haven't found anything, anywhere, that's any better.

I absolutely credit Melaleuca's unique vitamins and herbal tea for helping me avoid the flu and serious colds while remaining in an overall healthy condition these last two years, despite having diabetes.

For any problem that will respond to topical applications, such as scrapes, wounds, bites and cuts, I routinely use T36-C7™, Mela-Gel™, Problem Skin Lotion™ and Triple Antibiotic Ointment™. For sprains and sore muscles, I use Pain-A-Trate™.

I've proved to myself that it just makes real good sense to use products containing Melaleuca alternifolia oil. As I journey through my days and encounter surprise problems, I routinely turn to Melaleuca alternifolia oil to help solve them. From the stacks of letters on my desk and dining room table, I now know that many others have also found amazing success in treating their own problems when they've used the oil and products containing the oil.

So again: What have been your results, successes and even your disappointments when using Melaleuca alternifolia oil or products containing the oil? Please let me know!

THE FACTS: DIABETES AND MELALEUCA ALTERNIFOLIA OIL

As of this writing, an estimated 16,000,000 U.S. and Canadian citizens could have diabetes. However, the exact numbers having the disease can only be guess-estimated. Medical experts believe that at least half of all diabetics are unaware of their condition and will go undiagnosed until they have routine blood work, a physical examination, or until something unforeseen and unexpected happens.

If they're like me, they have ignored the common symptoms and are diagnosed only when an emergency situation happens. I didn't discover I was diabetic until the day after a wonderful cookie-tasting Christmas Day celebration when I nearly went into a coma. While I was developing the symptoms, I was not connecting them to diabetes. Maybe that's in part because of my original status - I am the only one in my extended family who's diabetic. Maybe I also was in a state of denial; I knew symptoms were happening, but they weren't so severe that I couldn't deal with them, or make excuses to myself about them. Then came Christmas and Bob and Marie's and Aunt Aleda's wonderful Scandinavian cookies and all the tempting treats. I yielded to temptation a few times during and after dinner - and the rest as they say, is now part of my medical history.

Attempting to estimate the numbers of American and Canadian citizens required to take daily insulin injections, or regular doses of oral medication, is however, somewhat easier. Extrapolating Canada's numbers with statistics from the American Diabetes Association and other sources, perhaps some 5,000,000 are now required to take single or multiple doses of insulin each day.

What is diabetes and what does it mean to be diagnosed diabetic?

These are questions often asked to those of us who are diabetic. Diabetes is a condition in which the pancreas stops producing insulin or the amount of insulin produced is insufficient. When either happens, it causes the blood's glucose level to become abnormally high. Since the body does not have the ability to store glucose, it is eliminated through excessive urination.

Combining this with constant thirst produces fatigue and weight loss.

High levels of sugar in the blood and urine impair the body's ability to fight infection. This can lead to problems including recurrent skin conditions, boils and carbuncles, tooth and gum problems, pneumonia and flu, and vaginal yeast infections. The initial signs of a potential problem in an undiagnosed diabetic will be a feeling of weakness, fatigue and unexplained weight loss. Weight loss is caused by cells starved for glucose that feed on the body's stored fat. In insulin-dependent diabetes, the fat breakdown process can lead to the production of acids that, if left untreated or undertreated, can ultimately result in coma and death.

Other symptoms of undiagnosed diabetes include blurred vision, increased appetite, and the sensation of tingling or numbness in the hands and feet. Symptoms will develop in all untreated insulin-dependent diabetics. However, they will only develop in about 30% of those having non-insulin-dependent diabetes. The two most common types of diabetes are type I and type II.

Type I diabetes develops rapidly. It is more severe and usually affects those under the age of 35. Insulin is used as a control measure. There is no known cure. Without regular insulin injections, the diabetic can lapse into a coma and die.

Those having type II diabetes are usually over the age of 40. The onset is often so gradual that many become aware of it only during routine medical examinations. Others are diagnosed after complications have already been detected. In type II diabetes, the pancreas produces small amounts of insulin. Diet and meal spacing are planned to help regulate carbohydrate intake, lower blood glucose levels and reduce excess weight. Where this treatment is not sufficient, anti-diabetic oral drugs that stimulate the pancreas are prescribed. Most with type II diabetes do not require insulin. However, there are thousands of type II diabetics (including this writer) that require daily injections of insulin.

Generally, people of color (Native Americans, Hispanics and African Americans) seem at significantly higher risks (when compared on a percentage basis) to developing diabetes than do those from other ethnic backgrounds. 10% of all African-Americans will one-day have the disease, the percentage jumps to 50% for American Indians, and one in three Hispanics will someday develop diabetes. Another surprising statistic is that one in five Japanese-Americans are at risk for developing diabetes.

Many diabetics face serious complications, particularly when their diabetes has not been well controlled or properly managed. These complications can include cataract development, damage to the retina, a higher risk of cardiovascular disorders, narrowing of the arteries, high blood pressure, damage to nerve fibers (or neuropathy) and kidney impairment.

A large variety of diabetic skin problems and infections start when blood sugar levels swing out of control. Those who are non-diabetic routinely fight off infection. However in a diabetic, when circulation is impaired, infection creates a greater risk. Even minor cuts and infections can create severe problems.

It is because of this potential for developing serious infection and gangrene that I am so excited about learning as much as possible, and sharing what I have learned about Melaleuca alternifolia oil. *When I was diagnosed as a diabetic, I thought I had ten years until I would go blind and they would cut off my feet. Through proper diet and vitamins, a program of steady (no more than a pound or two weekly) weight loss and exercise, and daily foot and leg inspections, I can still enjoy a healthy life. I absolutely advocate the use of Melaleuca alternifolia oil to treat cuts, skin breaks or abrasions. Now I sleep well at night knowing that my limbs will stay intact!*

When you first heard the words *"Melaleuca alternifolia oil"*, did you ever imagine this oil could offer a true life-and-limb-saving benefit for so many? ***Isn't it time you told someone who is diabetic about Melaleuca?***

People with diabetes have an increased risk for developing gum infections or periodontal disease. This condition is often more frequent and more severe in diabetics. It starts at an earlier age, often before the diabetic reaches 40. Periodontal infection can cause blood-sugar levels to drift out of control and play a major role in tooth loss. That is particularly important to diabetics, since dental problems, including poor or missing teeth, can make eating the right foods difficult, at best, and sometimes nearly impossible.

Gingivitis is the first stage of periodontal disease. Poor brushing and lack of flossing can lead to plaque buildup. Gums become red and infected leading to tooth decay. Melaleuca's Tooth Polish fights all types of gum and tooth problems. I have also used T36-C7™ on my sore gums, painting it on with either a finger or cotton swab. For those who do not have "store-bought teeth", active use of Melaleuca's Dental Floss™ is recommended.

T36-C7™ and T40-C5™ are effective in treating all types of cuts, abrasions, wounds, sores and skin injuries. One of the first published articles delineating the powers of the pure oil was in 1936 in *The Medical Journal of Australia*. This article described the effectiveness of Melaleuca alternifolia oil in successfully reversing a diabetic's gangrene. In the nearly six decades since that article appeared, countless numbers of diabetics have been helped by this miracle oil! *Isn't it time to put down this book and leap to your telephone to share the good news of Melaleuca alternifolia oil with a diabetic you know? I know for a fact they will appreciate your interest in helping them preserve and restore their good health!*

What Diabetics Should Know About Foot Care

In the United States, an estimated 4,000,000 diabetics are believed to encounter serious foot problems each year. Under the broad description of "foot problems", I include conditions such as wounds, blisters, sores, ulcers, abrasions, boils and nearly any type of skin condition that will not readily heal.

Neuropathy occurs in both type I and type II diabetes. It affects the nerves that connect the spinal cord to the muscles, skin, blood vessels and organs. Most often neuropathy affects the legs and feet. It causes symptoms such as numbness, burning, weakness, pain and tingling. Sensations start in the toes and move up the foot into the legs. Pain is often worse at night. Symptoms will depend primarily on which nerves are most affected. Sometimes nerve damage results in impotence, diarrhea, bladder infections and poor balance.

Since neuropathy causes the loss of feeling and sensation, cold and heat, pressure and even pain often go unnoticed. This means that sores and blisters, skin ulcerations and small cuts often go untreated. For this reason, diabetes literature advises diabetics to perform their own daily foot inspections. The injury, ignored, can lead to serious infection and possible gangrene, leading to one final treatment solution - amputation.

The American Diabetes Association reports that, ". . .15% of all [diabetics] will eventually develop foot ulcers. . .[that] frequently become infected and lead to amputation. 50 to 70% of all non-traumatic amputations occur in [diabetics]."

It's a proven fact that diabetics are more at risk for amputations since they're more at risk for developing serious foot infections. When a diabetic steps on a sharp object, the injury will often be undetected because prior nerve damage and poor circulation caused numbness and loss of feeling. An unnoticed or ignored injury is often the one that becomes infected. Even minor injuries or skin breaks have the potential to quickly become serious.

Anyone who's known to be at high risk for developing foot problems should be educated in the proper care and treatment of conditions affecting their feet. Learning to use Melaleuca alternifolia oil, and products containing the oil, will help heal most skin conditions. *However, the majority of physicians and primary care-givers I've encountered, still insist on prescribing strong drugs and lotions for foot care treatment. I just think they've closed their eyes to alternative remedies. Maybe I'm unusual, but most of the drugs I've had prescribed haven't worked as well for me as have Melaleuca's products. That's why, it's so important that every diabetic knows about, and understands, Melaleuca alternifolia oil and products containing the oil. And, when and how to use them.*

The American Diabetes Association encourages all diabetics to, "Wash your feet every day and carefully dry [the area] between the toes. Check feet and between the toes every day; look for blisters, cuts and scratches ... Before putting shoes on, [rub your fingers around the insides of each shoe to] check for pebbles or other objects ... that could hurt your feet ... Never walk barefoot ... Be careful when trimming toe nails; cut nails only straight across ... Good foot care can help prevent serious foot problems [from developing]."

The Association also cautions those who experience cold feet at night to wear an extra pair of stockings, instead of using a hot water bottle or heating pad; both may be too hot - and cause burns. It's also important that diabetics never soak their feet in hot water, since nerve damage may prevent them from determining the water's temperature. Nerve damage and loss of sensation or feeling aren't conditions that appear suddenly; more often, they come on so gradually that the person experiencing them is largely unaware - unless they're particularly *"tuned into their body parts"*. That's one reason why it's so important for all diabetics to make daily foot inspections.

Those with corns or calluses *must not* use products containing harsh chemicals, such as those sold over-the-counter in drug stores or pharmacies. (See Corn Removal Suggestions.)

Diabetics should avoid using any type of adhesive-backed tapes, strong chemicals or antiseptic solutions on their feet. Diabetics should avoid going barefoot. At home, wearing slippers or sneakers is important. Avoid wearing just stockings when "pattering" around the house. Never wear sandals or open toe shoes anywhere. Exercise particular caution when walking or sitting on hot beaches or on hot cement that surrounds outdoor swimming pools and hot tubs. Since diabetes causes nerve damage, many diabetics are unable to tell if the beach sand or paved areas are too hot for their feet. They can't determine temperature differences so they're unable to tell if the bottoms of their feet are just warm - or actually burning! Practicing basic caution will help diabetics avoid serious foot problems.

Many health care professionals believe amputations can be avoided by keeping diabetes under control, promoting and teaching the art of daily self-examinations, and using safe, natural products containing Melaleuca alternifolia oil. Recommended products include the Gold Bar™, Natural Spa & Bath Oil™, Anti-Bacterial Liquid Soap™, Problem Skin Lotion™, Body Satin™ Lotion, T36-C7™, T40-C5™, Mela-Gel™, Hand Creme™ and Triple Antibiotic Ointment™.

It's a safe assumption that *less than* 2% of America's diabetics have even heard of Melaleuca alternifolia oil and products containing the oil. Those of us who advocate the use of Melaleuca's products have our work "cut out" *(if you'll pardon an amputation term)* for us. We need to educate all diabetics, everywhere!

Diabetics face a greater risk in developing fungal infections, including itchy rashes in skin folds such as between the toes or under the arm. While other fungal condition treatments appear elsewhere in this book, I have added this here to remind all diabetics that they have a greatly increased risk of developing severe infections from conditions such as jock itch, athlete's foot, ringworm and vaginitis.

All of the evidence that I have gathered so far, indicates that Melaleuca alternifolia oil is more effective than any other treatment commonly available. I am confident that every sore, rash or skin problem I encounter can be eliminated by using products containing Melaleuca alternifolia oil.

My friends, Melaleuca alternifolia oil is indeed the good news in a small bottle! Please share what you have learned in these few pages with someone who needs to know. Their lives - and good health - could depend upon what you tell them.

For additional information on this subject, be sure to read "S.T. Clark's® Diabetes & Melaleuca Alternifolia Oil", that's also available through its publisher - Compton Park Companies, Inc. (222 Little Canada Road, Suite 175, Little Canada, MN 55117 - or 1-800-826-7932,),or Gaughan Fisch, Inc.

UNDERSTANDING
SUPER-ANTIOXIDANTS

The scientific name for antioxidants is Oligomeric Proanthocyanidins. Because the name is difficult to use in common language, we have, throughout this text, used such terms as: OPCs or OPC, antioxidants or super-antioxidants.

The importance of super-antioxidants is minimal. Particularly if you don't mind an early set of old-age symptoms such as heart disease, circulatory problems, and other deteriorations such as death. For most people the idea of aging and dying go hand-in-hand. One is a process leading to the other. But in the last quarter century, worldwide studies by scientists have shown that although we cannot end this, cannot stop the coming of the eternal footman - death - we can, perhaps, slow the arrival and enjoy good health for more time during the whole aging process.

We've all seen people who age faster than others. The scientific rationale for this points to many co-relating factors - genetic history, diet, exercise and others. One of the biological factors of aging is the process of oxidation. It creates "free-radicals" or damaged cells. These cells are pivotal to accelerating the body's decline into old age.

Since most of us over the age of 45 (I readily assume) wouldn't mind feeling healthier or twenty years younger, or even putting the biological brakes to our own age acceleration process, super-antioxidants become an important topic for discussion. One obvious reason is embedded in the name itself. If "oxidation" damages cells and promulgates old age, the term "anti-oxidant" should need little explanation.

At the most basic level, we need oxygen to live, to breathe. The unfortunate byproduct of this is that our bodies are sometimes inefficient in their use of that oxygen.

Think of a fire. If it burns cleanly, has few impurities, it will blow little dark smoke. However, if there are extraneous elements in what is burning, it can leave residue in the air (as my younger editors reportedly notice in their clothes and eyes during their camping forays) .

Similarly, if our bodies use oxygen inefficiently, they create smoke or free-radicals. In other words - damaged cells. Since we can't stop breathing without creating unpleasant side-effects, we have to improve the process of how our oxygen is utilized.

Now oxygen isn't all bad, but all of these excess damaged cells it leaves behind clutter the machine and don't allow the body to heal as easily. This is where super-antioxidants come in. What they actually do is eliminate the free-radicals that clog the system. Once the system is clear, the body can heal much more quickly and effectively.

OPCs, or antioxidants, occur naturally in many fruits and vegetables. Most studies show them as Vitamins A, C, and E, also noting that selenium seems to facilitate the healing process. Why bother to take super-antioxidants then?

One problem we humans seem to share is that, for most of us, we seldom eat enough fruits or vegetables to get OPCs in the amount our bodies actually need. If we have a busy schedule (we all do, don't we?), we frequently don't have time to stop off at the local grocery to unplug a few fruit loaves from aisle six. Let's say that on Monday afternoon we're in the mood for pizza for dinner. Who wants an apple and a bowl of peas when they have pepperoni on their agenda? On Tuesday, the neighbors invite us to their home for a fish dinner? Would you rather dine on a couple of bananas and some orange slices? Wednesday is a special day at the Senior Center where we help serve dinner and also stay for some roast pork and dressing, not to mention a few hands of cribbage. Would a plateful of fruit and vegetables seem a better choice? Thursday evenings usually have their own demands and then there's Friday and the weekend, and everyone knows there's no time there to consume a week's worth of natural antioxidants. Each of us usually has other priorities that appear and nearly always seem to get in the way of consistently doing what is sometimes termed - "best".

Another amazing circumstance to consider is that Melaleuca's super-antioxidant products are 20 to 50 times stronger than regular antioxidants. Taking several small pills daily is easier and more beneficial than consuming a full fruit basket over a week's period of time.

I can hear the wheels creaking in a few minds. And I can hear a lot of older folks saying that, well, I'm going to die anyway and I'd rather have fun while I do this living thing - even if it's for only a short time. True. Super-antioxidants are probably not going to keep anyone from eventually dying. But they ought to help make your ride better, allow you to stay more clear (mentally) and even prolong your good healthy years. The thing I really like about regularly taking super-antioxidants is that there's no rock and tether program to go through, or extensive paperwork to wade into. It's as simple as taking 2 to 6 very small pills once a day. That's not exactly a taxing regime.

All too often as our bodies age, we're faced with the realization that, oh gosh, we really are becoming our parents. *That realization is definitely a "Holy Cow" type of reality - and an added verification that now that we're approaching their age, perhaps they weren't so dumb or wrong, after all!* Statistically, there are not many of us who actually relish the idea of growing old, yet the fact remains that if we want to continue having birthday parties, we have to continue growing older.

For some, the introduction to super-antioxidants has come early; for others (like myself) antioxidants, we're just beginning to realize, are an important miracle product to help us fight the dragons of age and oxidation. I have found that by regularly taking OPCs, there is noticeable improvement in my personal health and in my diabetes control; you can list me under the "sold" category regarding belief in this product!

Antioxidants have long been recognized and promoted by many in both the scientific and medical communities. Oxidation occurs when almost anything is exposed to oxygen - iron rusts, a sliced apple or banana turns brown, food spoils and our bodies age and eventually wear out. Antioxidants work by fighting corrosion and tissue breakdown at the molecular level.

OPCs are both anti-aging and anti-disease. It's also no secret that antioxidants work to improve what can be termed "the innermost workings of the mind". They also uniquely help improve the lives of those having memory problems or those trying to live with the consequences of Alzheimer's Disease.

OPCs have become much more important to us than they were even in the past. Part of the reason for this can be traced to our current environmental conditions. The modern industrial environment we live in is conducive to creating a variety of harmful situations where our bodies are forced to produce many more free-radicals than what were generated in the past. In acknowledging this, it probably isn't too surprising that huge increases in the incidence of cancer, heart disease, allergies, diabetes, Alzheimer's and other illnesses can be the result of these potentially damaging factors exaggerated by conditions increasingly common to today's world. Such contributors could include pesticides, cigarette smoke, pollution, aluminum exposure, stress, sun radiation, food additives, carbons - and perhaps an entire host of other factors suspected, but not yet scientifically proven.

Antioxidants have been shown to help protect the body from the "natural" development of arthritis, heart disease, high cholesterol, some forms of cancer and a host of other non-infectious illnesses. They have also been shown to help reduce the effects of Parkinson's and Alzheimer's diseases. As mentioned above, while the primary benefit from taking antioxidants comes from neutralizing free-radicals, that benefit will often be evidenced by improved circulation, reduced inflammation, faster healing times, and a distinct slowing of the aging process.

Of course, most interesting to me are reports on diabetes. Many are finding, I have been told that over time their need for insulin is reduced. Since a great variety of diabetic-related secondary conditions involve circulatory problems, anything that can benefit and improve the body's circulation is absolutely important to the some 16,000,000 Canadian and U.S. diabetics.

Melaleuca has three antioxidant items in their product line. ProVex™ is a super-antioxidant made from grape seed extracts. Studies have shown that antioxidants taken from this source are more powerful, and plentiful, than ones secured from pine bark. ProVex Plus™ is similar to ProVex™ except that it contains some added herbal formulas to enhance your health.

The third product, Cell-Wise™, boasts an antioxidant formula, plus it contains all-natural Vitamin E, zinc, copper, selenium, and manganese. All of these helped convince me to use the aforementioned products. But, what really sealed my decision was that one day I walked down to the local health food store to have a look around. I noticed the various bottles of antioxidants and while I don't want to name brands or quote dollar-and-cent prices, I can tell you that retail on some exceeded $70 for just a 30-day supply. This is another thing I like about Melaleuca; shopping by phone is really easy. And considering costs, their prices are a real bargain. But insofar as quality is concerned, I absolutely believe Melaleuca's products are far superior to any other company's products available anywhere, from any source.

Who should take super-antioxidants? Well, to my way of thinking, anyone experiencing any non-infectious problem or illness, or anyone with a personal or family history of any of the conditions mentioned in the preceding three paragraphs should consider initiating (subject to the approval of their regular physician or primary care-giver) a regular program of super-antioxidant use. By consistently using these amazing OPCs in my own diabetic care program, I have come to realize that, for me, they work! Obviously, I urge you to investigate more fully how super-antioxidants can work for you, too.

*For additional information on the twin subjects of super-antioxidants **and** how to build and maintain a viable network marketing business, be sure to read "S.T. Clark's® Health to Wealth", available through Compton Park Companies, Inc. (222 Little Canada Road, Suite 175, Little Canada, MN 55117 - or 1-800-826-7932,),or through this publisher - Gaughan Fisch, Inc. .*

HOME SAFETY FACTS

A paper presented by a Vancouver consulting firm at the Indoor Air '90 Conference in Toronto, Ontario reportedly stated that because of household cleaners, housewives have a 55% higher risk of developing cancer than women who work outside the home.

What's the culprit? How about those dirty air filters on the furnace? That's a possibility that may contribute significantly to allowing even an immaculate home to become unhealthy. But how about all those household cleaners tucked away in closets, the laundry room and under the bathroom and kitchen sinks? Have you taken time to read their lists of ingredients? Do you really know what's in the products you're using to clean your home?

Fumes often escape from even tightly closed containers. This is why cleaning products have protective sealers that must be punctured or removed before the product can be used.

A September, 1991 Safety/Environmental Services message in the IBM Chemical Newsletter reported, "You are coughing, sneezing, and your eyes are irritated; you are suffering from chemical pollution - but you are far from industrial smokestacks and chemical plants. You're in your own kitchen! The EPA reported in 1985 that toxic chemicals found in every home, from drain cleaners to furniture polish, are *three times more likely to cause cancer* than airborne pollutants. The National Pollution Control Center estimates that the average home has approximately 62 different chemicals and that nearly 2,100,000 poisonings involving children six years and younger occur every year in the U.S.; older children and adults account for another 900,000 poisonings. No conscientious chemist would handle pesticides or even (household) cleaners without ventilation, goggles, and chemical gloves. Yet homemakers are advised by manufactures only to *'use caution'*. **The home is a complex chemical environment that contains many of the same chemicals that are known hazards in industry.** Workers are protected by the Right to Know law; the only real protection consumers have against hazardous chemicals is their own knowledge."

Those who fully investigate the cleaning products they have in their homes and who acknowledge the potential health risks in using them, will soon be shopping for alternatives. They also must find a safe method for the disposal of their harmful store-bought products. Some of these products actually are, I believe, as dangerous as placing a loaded gun within the easy reach of a 3 year old. This is a proper analogy to use for those intent on keeping very harmful chemicals within easy reach of any little creature living in, or visiting, their homes.

This is why we have converted our home to the safest products available. I am an admitted zealot in advocating that everyone switch their homes and lives to safer products. It stands to reason that natural products will be better than any products produced synthetically. For evidence of this, compare the air quality in a game preserve with that in an industrial dump. Some might think that this is a simple analogy, but those who believe their regular store-bought household cleaners are all okay, probably have not seriously considered the alternatives.

Here are some questions for those who have not yet switched their homes to safer products: Where do you want to live and spend your time? Where do you want your kids or grandkids to play? In cold weather when your doors and windows are closed, what do you want "stuck" in there with you?

You are to be congratulated if you have already switched your home's store-bought, harmful products to Melaleuca's safe products. Your decision will benefit you and your family and all those around you by not adding more pollutants to the common air.

Whenever you clean your home, clean with caution. Some believe the greatest danger coming from household cleaning products is in the possibility of a youngster drinking one of them. While that IS a danger, perhaps a greater danger is in poisons that can enter the body by inhaling or absorbing them through the skin. Vapors escape from even tightly closed containers and those products advocated to leave the home smelling bright and clean often pose the highest risk and danger.

Nancy Green Sokol, author of *"Poisoning Our Children"* (Noble Press) wrote, "Among the most toxic products (found in the home) are spray disinfectants or air fresheners which interfere with your ability to smell offensive odors by releasing a **nerve-deadening agent** or by coating your nasal passages with an oil film". Sokol also stated that "Indoor air pollution is a suspected culprit in sudden infant death syndrome, which will take about 5,000 U.S. lives this year. The incidence of SIDS is higher in the winter, perhaps because decreased ventilation in the cold months traps air indoors, where contaminants become concentrated. It's no coincidence that SIDS was recognized after the introduction of synthetic chemicals."

Many household products contain the same chemicals as those already included in strictly regulated industrial wastes. These also pose similar environmental problems. If you are in the process of converting your home to safer and healthier products, proper disposal of current household cleaners is important. In most areas, household garbage is taken to a landfill, incinerator or compost site. At landfills, buried household hazardous wastes can seep into ground water and contaminate drinking water supplies. At incinerators, household chemicals can cause fires or explosions, injuring workers and damaging facilities, and creating additional air pollution. At compost sites, household chemicals can contaminate the compost and restrict the ways in which the composted debris can eventually be used. You cannot get rid of your old household cleaners by flushing them or pouring them down the drain either. For safe disposal of *former* household cleaning products, contact your local pollution control agency for their recommendations.

Careless dumping of harmful household chemicals can, in time, hurt everyone. Dumping in storm sewers is like dumping directly into a lake or river. Dumping on the ground can mean eventual contamination of ground water and will affect drinking water wells. Dumping down the drain does not work either as many chemicals will pass through the system untreated. In a private septic tank, household cleaners dumped down the drain or flushed can block the very bacteria that make the system work. As a result, untreated sewage passes through soil, contaminating the ground water. This should be particularly important to anyone who has a private well and a private septic tank located anywhere near their home..

From the preceding paragraphs, can you estimate the amount of damage you may have inadvertently already caused yourself and your family from the year-after-year exposure to these hazards? Staggering when you think about it, isn't it? It proves again, that what you don't know sometimes really can hurt you.

How can you tell if the products in your home are unsafe? The best way is to read the product labels. Look for those "key" words that often are overlooked. These words include *"caution"* meaning a mild hazard. Or *"danger"* or *"warning"* indicating a significant hazard. But even more precautionary-type words appear on product labels that should warn anyone immediately of the danger in using them. For example, if the words *"flammable"*, *"combustible"*, or *"contains petroleum distillates"* appear, it means the product is considered to be hazardous because of it's flammability. The words *"contains acid"*, *"contains lye"*, or *"causes burns to skin"* indicate that a product is corrosive. The words *"harmful if swallowed"* mean the product is toxic and anything toxic is harmful or fatal if it is swallowed. Knowing what is written, and understanding precisely what the written words actually mean, is vital if you are to determine if your home is safe, or not safe.

These are reasons why I recommend buying alternative products that clean better, are safer, and do not need the "yuk" labels or warnings similar to those listed above. When you know the facts, decisions are always easier.

I will digress here to relate a story of how I put myself through school operating a mosquito and weed spraying business. Now, sometimes late at night when the rest of the house is asleep, I will go to the kitchen to make myself a cup of tea and just think about that. I lived with, sprayed and ingested DDT, 2-4-D and 2-4-5-T and other (now considered potent and extremely harmful) chemicals. This was the greatest summer time business I could have: I was young, free and knew I would live forever. It is only during the last 25 to 35 years that I have started to seriously think about whatever it is that remains unseen, that is still possibly crawling around somewhere, affecting the inside of my body. I n the last few years, I've have added pounds and given it a lot to crawl through - but if anything is there, it can probably be traced back to those three summers I worked to chemically defoliate and knock down trees, brush and small flying creatures. This is my serious side in telling you about dangers lurking in home chemicals, and dangers now acknowledged in pesticides and insecticides. I will let you know in 20 years if I am still around, what residual effects remain from those summers that enabled me to spend my winters in school and a lifetime pondering where another line of work could have taken me.

Reading the above paragraphs might help explain my passion in going to these extremes to warn you about the dangers of using traditional store-bought household chemicals and cleaners. If you are still using them, I think you are playing with a fire you can do something about. I do not think your risks are worth any possible return you could gain by having these harmful chemicals in your home. Do you?

However, if you insist on continuing to use harmful household chemicals and do not particularly care that the most toxic of all waste dumps is the one you sleep in at night, and the one your family calls home, then for the sake of your born and unborn heirs, learn how to use the products correctly.

To prevent accidental poisoning, always store hazardous products in areas where children and pets cannot get into them, such as in a locked cabinet outside the home (in a heated garage or shed). To keep products stable, find a cool, dry place that will not freeze. Make sure all caps and lids are as tightly sealed as possible. Always store in original containers. You might also consider putting the original container within a larger container having a sealable locking system. To limit your exposure risks, use harmful chemicals (if you absolutely insist on using them at all) in well-ventilated areas.

Do you live in a community that rallies to the cause when a company wants to create dumping grounds or more space for pollutants? That's good. Now, let's see what you can do to clean up your home and solve the problems that are far worse than what any new industry could bring to your community. They are worse because they are literally right under your nose. It is a proven fact that most homes contain more types of hazardous chemicals than exist in many factories. These harmful products contain components that weaken the immune systems.

Do you realize that many pollution control agencies list old cosmetics as hazardous waste? They are in the same category as latex paint, empty aerosols and water-based glue. Store-bought dandruff shampoos are some of the most toxic substances on the over-the-counter market. They can lead to a variety of health problems, particularly for anyone who suffers from asthma.

Products we bring into our homes can cause birth defects, headaches, burning eyes, skin rashes and a whole litany of problems we probably have yet to discover. We have yet to determine the long range genetic implications of these products and chemicals. *However, I would wager a small fortune that succeeding generations will not be mentally helped by what we have chosen to do in our generation. And, I guarantee you, they will not be impressed that a grandparent or two (a few times or more removed) tried to save some pennies making decisions that ultimately resulted in costing them their ability to reproduce anything that looks reasonably human. This contamination has spread from mere theory to reality. Friends, we are sitting on an ecological time bomb.*

Are you aware that many household mold and mildew cleaners contain formaldehyde? I have heard that some of the more popular laundry cleaners and even common brands of dish soap, also contain formaldehyde. If you wear soft contact lenses, vapors rising from solvents and pesticides can attach to the lens and do long-term damage to your eyes. *Maybe wearing glasses isn't so bad, after all.* Some spot removers contain chemicals that cause confusion, weakness and fatigue. Warning labels only tell the immediate effects from exposure. They do not list the potential long-term health risks.

Children face a greater risk from harmful household chemicals. They breathe faster, weigh less and have more fatal poisoning accidents. If you have had your carpets professionally cleaned lately, do you know the cleaning ingredients that were used? Many commercial carpet shampoos contain respiratory irritants. The reason they tell you to open the windows is not just to allow the carpeting to dry, but also because of the toxic chemicals in the solutions they use. I could extend this chapter by another 20 pages describing what can go wrong in your home from using products that will negatively affect your health and that of your family, but by this time you should have some ideas on how to make your home safer.

So, isn't it time you switched to products that are proven to be safer for you, your family, pets, AND the environment? Taking care of your family means being in control of some of the decisions that can affect their health, well-being and day-to-day lives. By using products containing effective Melaleuca alternifolia oil, you will be taking some giant steps in making your home the safe haven you planned for all those you love and are responsible for nurturing.

It is now time to change words into action. If you have not already changed your home, now is the time folks. Now IS the time.

TESTIMONIALS

"My husband and brother-in-law own a small restaurant and when they come home at night, the front of their shirts are usually oil-stained from the fryers and grill. I just heard about MelaPower™ and started using it several weeks ago. I have tried many other cleaners and found none could match the power of MelaPower™. This product sure has the right name. It truly is powerful!" **-L.H., Minnesota**

"After using Tub 'N Tile™ cleaner and Sol-U-Guard™ disinfectant cleaner in my shower, we no longer have mildew problems. I tried giving all my old harsh cleaning products to a neighbor, but she wanted to know why I was doing that. When I told her I had switched to something safer, she wouldn't take my stuff. Now she's buying products from Melaleuca, too. We still have this box of stuff to give away and are looking for ideas on how to get rid of it." **-D.L., Minnesota**

"Since converting our home to Melaleuca products, our entire family has noticed that none of us are bothered any longer by chemical sensitivity caused by bought cleaners we once purchased, stored in our home and used. The only times we get headaches and nausea from chemicals now, are either when we visit friends (who won't switch to Melaleuca's safe products), or when we're exposed to the commercial stuff at our local discount grocery store." **-C.S., Arizona**

"Your book offers the most readable and in-depth explanations of why Melaleuca alternifolia oil is so effective in treating so many problems. Please send me another 100 copies (the first 100 sold out before my meeting had even started); I want to make sure that each member of my downline team has their own copy. With this book, I'm sure that everyone who reads it will finally get the full picture and understand how valuable Melaleuca oil is to their lives and their financial future. S.T. has a unique gift for writing and for bringing us what we need to know about Melaleuca. He has a unique story-telling ability that kept me interested in turning the pages rather than skipping around to see "what fit". I think that all Melaleuca-people need to read this book and then pass their copy - or another one - on to their personal enrollees, family and friends. Thank you for publishing the book. And thank S.T. for writing it, too!" **-W.E., Florida**

Assembling An Emergency Care Kit

I believe that one of the most responsible things I can do for my family is to prepare for any contingency. Part of my preparations include having available those items that may be critical in the event of an emergency.

After thinking about what I would do in the event of something unforeseen, I decided to assemble an emergency-care kit. After converting our home to Melaleuca products, I soon realized that our old first-aid kits were out-dated and incomplete. To me, an emergency-care kit is an essential form of insurance. Having something not needed is far more important than needing something and not having anything available.

This led me to the decision that if I was to be the "protector" of my family, then I would by necessity need a basic emergency-care kit stocked with Melaleuca products. Soon into my project, I realized that one kit would be insufficient, so I decided to assemble several. Now I have kits for my home, car, truck, boat and office.

Perhaps I have packed in too much stuff, or maybe there is something I should have included that is missing. I figure the kits contain a reasonable number of products that will treat all common emergencies, at least until professional help arrives.

My generic supplies include: a flashlight with new batteries, two candles, dry matches, glass thermometer, a pair of tweezers, small and large sharp scissors, bulb syringe, an assortment of bandages including ace and compression, tourniquet, some *breathable* sterile gauze and one bottle each of aspirin, acetaminophen and antacid. No kit would be complete without a bottle of Ipecac syrup that will induce vomiting in the event of a poisoning. I have also included a roll of paper tape, rather than adhesive. Diabetics should avoid using adhesives because of potential damage to the skin when removing the tape.

Since I'm diabetic, my kits contain items that pertain to my diabetes. This means I include extra supplies such as insulin, needles, test strips, glucose tablets, sugar packets and cotton. If someone in your family is on a particular medicine, ask your pharmacist to package several smaller bottles; then place at least one in each kit. (Be sure to watch the expiration dates and replace supplies as often as necessary.) This way, in an emergency, medication will continue uninterrupted.

While I'm updating this in Minnesota in the late-autumn of 1995, my thoughts go to those who survived the calamities of the past several years. With earthquakes and fires in the west, and floods in the midwest and south, hurricanes pounding the southern coasts, temperatures exceeding normal highs most of the summer and creeping down to record lows in winter months, it truly seems that no large area of the U.S. or Canada was spared from some natural calamity. Each year produces more rounds of floods, earthquakes, record cold waves and record heat/humidity, tornadoes and windstorms, fires and mishaps.

We share many common conditions as human beings including the unknown that waits for us all as we plod through our days. We cannot really forecast when we will need to grab our emergency-care kit and race for higher ground, an underground shelter or appropriate cover or protection. Because of the unknown that might one day happen, it is a wise person that follows the Boy Scout rule and decides to "Be Prepared!"

A copy of this book has been added to each kit I assembled. Many of the remedies included here were first detailed in a treatment notebook I wrote for my kits.

In each emergency care kit, I include these Melaleuca products:

T36-C7™
T40-C5™
Melaleuca's Liquid Soap™
Hot Shot™
Problem Skin Lotion™
Body Satin™ Lotion
Sol-U-Mel™
Mela-Gel™
Sun-Shades 9™ and 15™
Access Bars™
Sustain Drink Mix™
Pain-A-Trate™
Triple Antibiotic Ointment™
Nature's Cleanse™
Several tea bags of G'Day™ Melaleuca Herbal Tea.

I use sample size portions of many products and also include bottles of Sol-U-Mel™ and Tough 'N Tender™ in several of the kits. I believe that each item listed may be important, since I have no idea what problem or calamity may one day occur. I also consider each a "Melaleuca-standard".

However, this list of inclusions should be used only as a guide. Anyone who assembles a kit should place in it those items that pertain to their own situation. For example, if someone in your family cannot live without a Gold Bar™, by all means include several sample size bars.

It's important that each member of your household understand the kit's purpose. It isn't a backup supply to be used when regular supplies are depleted. Doing that will only insure that your kit will be incomplete when and if it's needed. I've learned that if something is borrowed, it usually isn't replaced; so frequently check your inventory.

Include a small notebook to record your family members' brief medical histories. Write the name, telephone number and address of physician, dentist, pharmacy with prescription numbers, dates of past surgeries and hospitalizations, immunizations, allergies and lists of ongoing medical problems. Hopefully, the better prepared you are, the less likely you will be to need your emergency care kit.

These emergency kits are an ideal and practical gift for birthdays, weddings, anniversaries, retirements, going-away parties, the holidays, and for young people going off to college. Before you assemble one to give away, make sure you have one or two for your own home. *One never knows what lies ahead or is coming around the bends in the roads of their tomorrow's. So become the good scout - and be prepared!*

TESTIMONIALS

"I know that during pregnancy, a woman's gums can become swollen, inflamed and will bleed easily. As a former dental hygienist, I am aware that this can lead to serious problems. At my last dental appointment, when I was 6 months pregnant, my hygienist asked what I was doing differently. My gums were very healthy and had significantly improved since my last visit. I told her about Melaleuca's Tooth Polish. Since I have been regularly using these products, I have had the best check-ups ever. Now both my hygienist and dentist use Melaleuca, too." **-D.H., Minnesota**

"I once was bothered by a fluid build-up around my ears that resulted in my frequently having terrible ear aches. A friend suggested I use Pain-A-Trate™ followed by Problem Skin Lotion™ as a topical rub on the affected areas (being careful to not drip the products into my ear canals). After you've suffered from pain for awhile, any solution anyone offers has to be seriously considered. I am really amazed at my results from using these two products. I think one reason both worked so well is that they really tend to move in below the skin level and stimulate the blood vessels, which to my understanding helps promote healing. From now on, I plan to always keep a supply of this amazing oil close by." **-G.G., Idaho**

"Here's a solution to a problem that I'll bet no one else has probably sent in: I was having a problem with a skin condition on the back of my head and couldn't seem to figure out anything that would work to heal it with the products I had on hand. Since I had about half a bottle of Nature's Cleanse and no T36-C7™ or Melaleuca shampoo, I used what I had. Imagine my surprise! After just two "treatments", the condition disappeared - never (it's been 3 months) to return. It probably isn't amazing to you since I'll bet you're receiving all kinds of testimonials from all sorts of different people about results they're obtaining using Melaleuca's products - but, it sure surprised and impressed me! The only question now is, do I get a "complimentary copy of the first edition of The Great Melaleuca Fact Book that this appears in?" **-M.S., Minnesota**

Editor's Note: You bet! A copy of this book has been sent to you. Now can we give a copy of the next edition to anyone else? Does anyone else have any other success stories using Melaleuca products?

CLEANING FACTS

Melaleuca alternifolia oil is an effective solvent and natural cleaner that dissolves stains and resins. It is an ideal ingredient in cleaning products and is proven effective when used in these applications:

wall paper removal

paint removal

drapes

fly control

tires and wheels

garden stained hands

hot tubs and saunas

blood stains

broiler pans

floors

counter tops

crayon

dishes

dusting

fruit and vegetable washing

furniture

waste baskets

gum

rugs

laundry

lipstick

fungi, mold and mildew

rust

upholstery

windows

diaper pails

china stains

appliance cleaning

awnings

blinds

automobile - exterior and interior

bathrooms

toilets and sinks

mirrors

copper and brass

fireplaces

ceilings and walls

cutting boards

scuff and heal marks

doors

fine washables

garage floors

garbage cans

grass stains

ink

jewelry

odor elimination

roaster pans

mud

tile

water spots

piano keys

computers & office equipment

boats

grass stains	shoes
snowmobiles	motorcycles
bicycles	tick removal
tubs	

A previous section told how to assemble an emergency care kit. I believe it's just as important to also have assembled a reasonable arsenal of household cleaning weapons - products to have on hand when and where needed. Maintaining a supply allows you to effectively and safely clean all areas of your home.

One of the first things we did when converting our house to Melaleuca products was to purchase a supply of spray bottles, a good squeegee, sponges, several terry cloth towels, a new broom and a better step stool.

Having just attended one of Wisconsin's better county fairs, I did not need the vacuum - but it was a deal I knew I could not turn down. So, as I am writing this, I am looking at this enormous cleaning machine having more attachments than what I can reasonably figure out.

Now that preceding sections have explained some of the environmental and health reasons to consider when buying cleaning products, maybe a breakdown of costs-per-use for Melaleuca's concentrated cleaning products should be included. I have estimated the costs for cleaning different areas of my home and can now report the following:

TOILET BOWL CLEANER
Tub 'N Tile™ $0.05 per use

WINDOW CLEANER
Tough 'N Tender™ $0.0004 per ounce
(I pay $0.01 for 32 ounces. One quart
of concentrate equals 400 quarts of cleaner.)

BATHROOM CLEANER
Tub 'N Tile™ $0.05 per ounce

ALL-PURPOSE CLEANERS, MISC.
Tough 'N Tender™ $0.0008 per ounce
(This is 2.5 cents per quart. One quart of
concentrate equals 192 quarts cleaner.)

Disinfectants & Deodorizers

Sol-U-Mel™ $1.43 per ounce
(However, usually only a capful
is used in most cleaning recipes.)

Floor Cleaner

Tough 'N Tender™ $0.0008 per ounce
(Or, just 2.5 cents per quart. One quart of
concentrate equals 192 quarts cleaner.)

Automatic Dishwashing Cleaner

Diamond Brite™ $0.10 per ounce
(Or, just $0.05 per use with soft water.)

If you're a wise consumer, you will probably want to do your own cost comparisons. Compare the costs-per-use with products purchased in your local grocery or area discount store. *Personally, I think you are wasting your time and that you do not stand a proverbial snowball's chance of proving store-bought products are cheaper to use than Melaleuca! Then again, it is your time to spend. So, go for it! Just let me know how you come out!*

For comparison purposes, consider a quart of Melaleuca's all-purpose cleaner Tough 'N Tender™. It costs about $4.80 (plus tax and shipping). But, because it's concentrated, it produces 192 quarts of an effective cleaner. This reduces the effective cost to under three cents per quart. How does this compare with the "store-bought" cleaners you have purchased? Or with any other all-purpose cleaners available anywhere else?

Now, I'm not as big a fan of cleaning as I am of saving money. Maybe that's in part due to some frugal Norwegian ancestors who wore their long underwear as a protector against winter cold and summer heat. At least it was cheaper than buying short underwear to wear for just a few months. So spending three cents for a quart of the best and safest cleaning product available certainly makes sense to me. And I even wear short underwear.

Some may find my suggested chore remedies won't work as well for them as I've suggested they work for me. That's okay really, since conditions always seem to differ. We each work with our own chore problems and we each work within our own environments. For example, we don't have a water softener; those with softeners should use less product than what I suggest. Some claim they obtain excellent results when quantities are reduced by 50%. That's why I urge you to experiment with product quantities to determine what works best for you in your own situation.

TESTIMONIALS

"One of my horses was injured recently when it tangled with an electric fence. The injury burned her hair on part of her chest and created a swelling that was nearly a foot in diameter. I made a mixture of 2 tablespoonfuls Sol-U-Mel™, 1 teaspoonful Natural Spa & Bath Oil™ and a few drops of T40-C5™ to rub into the swollen area. The next day the swelling was down considerably. I then washed the injured area with a capful of Anti-Bacterial Liquid Soap™ combined in a 5-gallon bucket of warm water. I washed her down well and then after drying, I applied Pain-A-Trate™ to the site. The swelling continued to decrease, and the injury stayed confined to the one area without spreading. In about a week, the injured site was vastly improved."

-E.T., California

"I just wanted to tell you how blessed our family is now that we have discovered Melaleuca alternifolia oil. I know that we still need our doctors, but now we think of Melaleuca products first when faced with any new medical crisis. We are truly fortunate we have Melaleuca, our doctors and our family's improving health."

-J.R., Minnesota

"When my two cats both developed a mite problem on their chins, they rubbed the skin raw with their continued itching. I read the Melaleuca literature and decided to treat each of them with an application of T36-C7™. Before I had a chance to apply some Mela-Gel™, they disappeared somewhere in the house. But, the next day they came purring back, no longer scratching; their once open wounds were already starting to heal. I then applied a thin coating of Mela-Gel™, which they liked almost as much as the pure Melaleuca oil. By the third or fourth day, the skin was well on its way to being healed, so I applied Triple Antibiotic Ointment™ several times daily and continued with applications of either Mela-Gel™ or the ointment for the next week. I have to say - maybe even shout - how much I value Melaleuca products! I don't know what the vet would have charged, but I'm sure I saved money using Melaleuca products. However, when it comes to taking care of my cats, the actual expense or savings isn't as important as my knowing that my animals are in their best physical condition possible."

-Mrs. T.B., Rhode Island

CHORE LIST WITH SUGGESTED REMEDIES

The following suggested remedies for some of the more frequent household chores, are based upon what works best in my home and in the homes of those I know who are using Melaleuca's cleaning products. There will be differences in cleaning results achieved; this can be attributed to the amounts of product used, mineral content of water, temperature, hardness (or softness) of water, degree of cleaning skill required to perform the necessary chore, ability of the person "selected" to accomplish the chore, age of the stain or task (how long was it "put off"?) and other known and unknown, but often similar, contributing factors.

I have learned that when using Melaleuca's concentrates, sometimes less product used creates the best results. Most store-bought cleaners can't claim the results routinely achieved by Melaleuca's products. Plus Melaleuca's cleaners provide amazingly low cost-per-use results. *That fact alone would really have appealed to some of my ancestors.*

Writing from my home in Minnesota gives me many insights; however, it doesn't allow me to determine what may or may not work best for you in your own home. Remedies suggested are based on results achieved from conditions as they were found at the time the actual chore was performed.

Maybe you should think of these remedies as a map to a wonderful landscape; if you want to live where you can look out at a mountain range, or an open harbor, or a wooded lakeshore, your only decision will be trying to best determine a plan to get there. I believe that Melaleuca's products provide the truest road to a safe, near-perfect home. And while many roads lead to this beautiful place of dreams briefly envisioned, some roads will take you in circles -more than I probably have just done in this paragraph's opening sentences. All of these words though, serve as your introduction to the alphabetical assembly known here as the Chore List With Suggested Remedies section of "S.T. Clark's® Great Melaleuca Fact Book."

Air Freshener:

Combine 2 to 3 capfuls Sol-U-Mel™ with 8 ounces water in a spray bottle. Spray the air to make it fresh smelling and safe. Many commercial fresheners actually deaden your sense of smell rather than eliminating odors. Check the ingredient differences in Melaleuca's products and the stuff that is commonly available from your local grocery store. Then decide what products you want to expose your family to before you buy. In the beginning and in the end, it is your buying decision.

Aluminum Utensils:

Most people have few if any aluminum pots, pans and even utensils remaining in their homes. *There is a reason one sees so much aluminum in garage sales and I don't think it has much to do with the public's demand for these products.* **As a word of caution:** Never wash or soak anything that is aluminum, including old kitchenware and utensils, with other dishes, pots or pans. Aluminum can be very harmful and even toxic to your own and your family's health. If you still have some old aluminum pots and pans, isn't now a good time to safely dispose of them?

Appliances:

Always unplug any electrical appliance prior to cleaning it. When cleaning kitchen appliances, I generally prefer to use 1 teaspoonful Tough 'N Tender™ and 1 capful Sol-U-Mel™ combined in a 32 ounce spray bottle filled with water. After spraying, I have found it works best if you allow the spray to remain on the appliance for a minute or so before wiping off. This is an effective and safe cleaner that seems to inhibit future dust and dirt buildups.

For heavier cleaning chores and to remove kitchen grease, add 4 ounces MelaMagic™ and 1 capful Sol-U-Mel™ to a gallon of water. As a spray, I double the quantities of both MelaMagic™ and Sol-U-Mel™. Never use abrasive cleaners or scouring pads on appliances.

Judith, an award-winning poet who lives down the street from us, is the only person I know who cleans the outside of her Melaleuca bottles upon delivery. She also is probably the most fastidiously clean, cleaning person I know. She uses ClearPower™ for all her appliance and kitchen cleaning chores, and claims it is always effective in wiping out both grease and grime. *Good grief, how can **they** possibly form in her house? She doesn't seem to do anything but clean. Judith has written a poem about her cleaning experiences. However due to lack of space, I will forego publishing it here. But, maybe in the next edition…*

AUTOMOBILES:

Have you tried Tough 'N Tender™ in your windshield washer tank yet? If you are tired of paying nearly a dollar a gallon for store-bought windshield cleaner that consists mainly of some blue-colored water, a splash of chemical, printed label and a non-recyclable bottle, you have to try this recipe! Just add *3-5 drops* Tough 'N Tender™ to every 4 ounces water. After just a tankful, I am sure you will agree that **this** is "an amazingly adequate" solution for dirty windshields!

Mix 1 capful Sol-U-Mel™ and 2 ounces MelaMagic™ in a 16 ounce spray bottle and fill with water. Use this solution for cleaning under the hood. After spraying on, hose off dirt and grime. Have you tried cleaning whitewall tires using 2 to 3 tablespoonfuls Diamond Brite™ dissolved in a cup of water? For dirty tires, make a paste of Diamond Brite™ and Tub 'N Tile™. Brush on and rinse off.

To effectively wash your car, add just 1 tablespoonful Tough 'N Tender™ to a gallon of water. Wet the car first, then sponge this on and hose down to rinse. ClearPower™ works well on your car's windows and interiors. Follow the directions printed on the bottle.

AWNINGS

Use 1 tablespoonful Tough 'N Tender™ for this chore. We have only two awnings and both seem to pick up all the season's dirt and grime. 1 tablespoonful in a gallon of water is all that's needed. Sometimes, I also add 1 capful Sol-U-Mel™, then sponge the awnings before rinsing. This works every time without leaving streaks or water spots.

BABY WIPES:

This is a cost-effective method for making safe baby wipes. Combine 1 teaspoonful Sol-U-Mel™ OR 1 capful Nature's Cleanse™ to 1 capful Natural Spa & Bath Oil™, 1/4 teaspoonful Tough 'N Tender™ and 2 cupfuls water. Use a kitchen knife to cut a roll of paper towels in half. Remove the cardboard roll from the center and begin pulling the towels from the center. Place in a plastic container and pour the solution over. Replace the lid and cut a "star" in the center. You can then pull the towels through. A plastic 1/2 gallon frozen yogurt container seems to work the best.

I am not handy, but even I have been able to build this. These wipes actually work. My only problem is that since we have no baby in the house, I have had to find some other uses for my "baby wipes".

BAR-B-QUE GRILLS

I use a tooth brush (but any small firm brush will work as well) to apply

Tough 'N Tender™ undiluted to the grill. Allow it to stand for several minutes before rinsing off. If the burned-on-grit is really extensive, use 1 ounce MelaMagic™ combined with 8 ounces water. Brush on and leave alone for several minutes before rinsing off.

BATHROOMS:

30+ years ago, I lived in New York City for one summer. While there, I met a couple who were "johnny-cleaners" going from bar to bar cleaning those horrid public rest rooms. Since then, I have never met anyone else who actually "wanted " to clean bathrooms. Well, this is the '90s and some things do change. Even I can be corrected in my beliefs.

I was surprised to hear that my friend Dave discovered Melaleuca's cleaning products' effectiveness. His wife Barb tells the story that upon opening his Melaleuca delivery, Dave took the first bottle of Tub 'N Tile™ and headed upstairs to their new master bathroom's shower. Lines of mold were already blackening the new tile's grouting. Barb reported that Dave spent ten minutes laughing and giggling while cleaning his bathroom tiles and himself. *Now whenever I hear profuse giggling up or down my street, well - I just sort of figure another neighbor has probably discovered how to clean some mold-stricken bathroom tile.*

Bathroom Bacteria: Sol-U-Guard™ kills bathroom bacteria. *I think it really would work perfectly for anyone in the commercial johnny-cleaning business, too.* For proper germicidal cleaning action, be sure to thoroughly wet the surface with Sol-U-Guard™ and water. After spraying, let stand for 15 minutes. This assures proper germicidal action. Some recommend adding 5 to 6 ounces Sol-U-Guard™ per gallon of water for an effective one-step cleaning and disinfecting aid. Depending upon the surface to be cleaned, use 8 to 16 ounces Sol-U-Guard™ per gallon of water.

Bathroom - Hard Water Spots: Add 2 tablespoonfuls Sol-U-Mel™ and 2 tablespoonfuls Tub 'N Tile™ to a quart of water. Spray on to remove hard water spots. I think you will discover that this will wipe out fungus, mold and mildew while it cleans, shines and polishes. Never use Tub 'N Tile™ on genuine marble surface.

Bathroom - Mildew & Mold: For mildew control, add 5 to 6 ounces Sol-U-Guard™ and 1 to 2 capfuls Sol-U-Mel™ per gallon of water. Wet the surfaces and use a small brush to scrub the mildew growth away. Rinse with clean water. If there is a build up of mildew and mold, apply Tub 'N Tile™ full strength. Spray on and let stand a few minutes before rinsing off. If it dries, just re-spray and wait less time before rinsing off. This also is an excellent mixture to use when cleaning mold and mildew off bathroom shower curtains.

Bathroom - Toilet: Use 1 tablespoonful Tub 'N Tile™ in a 16 ounce spray bottle to coat around the inside rim of the toilet. If stains are heavy, use full strength. Allow this to remain on before scrubbing with a toilet brush. I also use Diamond Brite™ as a bowl cleaner, dissolving 1 teaspoonful first in a cup of hot water. Pour into toilet and let stand for several minutes before brushing clean.

My friend Dennis refurbishes old houses and small apartment buildings. He uses this mixture to clean the old toilets and bathroom fixtures: 1 ounce Sol-U-Guard™ combined in a 16 ounce spray bottle of water. He turns the toilet's water off and flushes the tank to empty the bowl. Dennis then sprays a heavy amount of the mixture in the tank and bowl, making sure he has doused the bowl's underside rim, the exterior and round the toilet base and floor. Dennis then waits a few minutes before turning the water back on and flushing. He can then rinse all exterior areas with a damp sponge before wiping dry.

Bathroom - Toilet Bowl Cleaner & Rust Remover: This is a low cost-per-use effective toilet bowl cleaner and rust remover. Use a small margarine container and punch holes in the lid. Add a rock to the container. Then fill with Diamond Brite™ and a small amount of water. Place in toilet tank. This is an economical and safe toilet bowl cleaner.

BLEACH SUBSTITUTE:

Have you tried adding Diamond Brite™ to white clothes? The results warrant a definitive "WOW!" Dissolve 1 to 2 tablespoonfuls Diamond Brite™ in hot water, add laundry and MelaPower™ to clean as usual. Sometimes, I add 1 tablespoonful Diamond Brite™ to colored clothes, providing they are colorfast. I am amazed at how bright some of my older clothes now look. If you have some badly stained clothes, try soaking them overnight in a washer, tub or bucket of water to which you have added 1 to 2 tablespoonfuls Diamond Brite™.

BLINDS:

Cleaning blinds is best done in a flat open area. *Such as North Dakota or Montana. Or Texas.* But seriously, remove blinds and open to their full length after placing them on a tarp, blanket or plastic sheet. Use 1 tablespoonful Tub 'N Tile™ in a 16 ounce spray bottle filled with water. Liberally spray directly on the slats. Rinse well and repeat process on the reverse side of the slats. Allow to dry thoroughly before attempting to rehang.

BLOOD STAINS:

Blood is always difficult to remove from carpeting or clothes. Luckily, in our home, we have not had an injury or the necessity that requires *"knowing"* how to remove spilled blood. But, others who have been less fortunate tell me they have used Pre-Spot™ to attack the stain. Just spray Pre-Spot™ on the affected area of carpeting and place a damp clean towel over the stain. Press gently to blot, as you frequently change the area of the towel that is used. Always try to blot with a clean portion of the towel. Re-spray Pre-Spot™ and blot as necessary.

For clothing with blood stains, use Pre-Spot™. Apply it directly on the stain. Wait a few minutes for it to work in, then gently rub fabric against fabric followed by rinsing in cold water. For washing blood-soiled clothes, use 1/8th of a cup MelaPower™ and 1 to 2 capfuls Sol-U-Mel™.

BOATS:

We have an aluminum fishing boat that stays tied to the dock most of the summer. In the fall and sometimes when being ultra-inspired before autumn, I will drag the boat up on shore, turn it over and clean the bottom residue. This also empties out most of the leaves, old bait and dried food left-overs from under the seats or tucked under the anchor rope. I have found that mixing 1 ounce MelaMagic™ with 8 ounces water (and the requisite 1 capful Sol-U-Mel™) is the best cleaner for this chore. To clean the boat's inside, use MelaMagic™ or Tough 'N Tender™, spraying it on and wiping off the dirt and built-up scuff marks. Our neighbor, Jim, uses a slightly different variation to clean his boat. He combines 1 ounce Tub 'N Tile™ with 3 ounces water and 1 capful Sol-U-Mel™. After letting this soak, Jim washes the boat off using 2 tablespoonfuls Tough 'N Tender™ to a gallon bucket of water and then hosing it down.

Whichever method you try, what is most important is that you can safely clean your boat and outdoor equipment and furnishings using any of Melaleuca's cleaning products. There is no worry about contaminating the ground, lake or river water.

BRASS:

Have you seen what Tub 'N Tile™ will do to tarnished brass? All you need do is spray it on and wipe the grit and black tarnish away. It is really quite amazing and so simple, too.

BROILER:

After baking or broiling anything, and even before sitting down to enjoy the latest culinary adventure, I will run some warm water into the broiler or oven pan and add a couple squirts of undiluted Tough 'N Tender™. If I have really outdone myself and the roast has produced some unbelievably fine residue, I use 1 part MelaDrops™ mixed with 8 parts water to spray the pan.

After dinner and after the last cup of coffee has gone south, I know the broiler pan can be easily rinsed clean. *I credit Tough 'N Tender™, MelaMagic™ and MelaDrops™ as the three principal reasons behind my success as a chef, and my success in creating harmony (despite the mess I "conjure" up in the kitchen) at home.*

BUMPER STICKER REMOVAL:

When the campaign is over, how do you remove all traces of whom you supported? Well, I have a post-election "solution" for you. Apply either Sol-U-Mel™ undiluted, or Tough 'N Tender™ undiluted. The old bumper stickers should disappear in only one application.

CARPET CLEANER (MACHINE MIX):

When cleaning any carpeting, FIRST check the color fastness before using any cleaning product. After determining that the carpeting can be safely cleaned, combine 1/2 cupful MelaPower™ with 1/4 cupful MelaMagic™ and 2 capfuls Sol-U-Mel™ in 3 gallons of water. This is an effective cleaning solution that really works. Plus, it is safe to use around small children and pets. There is no need to open windows and doors for ventilation when cleaning with Melaleuca products. When using a carpet cleaning machine, use 1 capful Sol-U-Mel™ and 1 capful Tough 'N Tender™. If you have soft water, reduce the amount of cleaners used by at least 50%. Rinse carpeting well after steam cleaning or shampooing. If any cleaning residue remains, it will attract dust and you will be repeating your carpet cleaning chores more often.

CARPET SPOTS:

In a 16 ounce spray bottle, I combine 1 teaspoonful Tough 'N Tender™ and 1 capful Sol-U-Mel™ and fill the bottle with water and shake to mix. For grease spots on carpeting, I've had excellent results using a solution of 1 ounce MelaMagic™ combined with 7 to 8 ounces water.

CEILINGS:

For general cleaning tasks: Mix 1 teaspoonful Tough 'N Tender™ in a 16 ounce spray bottle of water or add 1 tablespoonful Tough 'N Tender™ to a gallon bucket of water. You can boost the disinfectant ability if you add 1 capful Sol-U-Mel™ to either the spray or bucket.

For heavy duty cleaning: Use 1 part MelaMagic™ with 8 parts water. Add 1 capful Sol-U-Mel™. This is ideal for all heavy-duty cleaning chores. All-purpose Tough 'N Tender™ spray seems to also work well when Sol-U-Mel™ has been added.

For disinfecting: Add 1 ounce Sol-U-Guard™ and 1 capful Sol-U-Mel™

to a 16 ounce spray bottle filled with water. I would recommend that with any cleaning and disinfecting chore, you start by using less product concentrate, and then slowly increase the amounts of product used until you have a solution that will be effective in dealing with your own chore. Keep in mind that Melaleuca products are concentrated. Only small amounts are necessary to yield large results.

CHEWING GUM:

If the chewing gum is in fabric, remove all the "excess" gum you reasonably can before applying undiluted* Sol-U-Mel™. Then rub fabric against fabric - if possible. If the chewing gum is in carpeting, first remove what you can. Then use a toothbrush or a cloth dampened with full strength* Sol-U-Mel™, using that to help you bring out and clean the area affected. *ALWAYS check the color-fastness of the carpeting, clothing or textile you intend to clean BEFORE applying undiluted Sol-U-Mel™ or any cleaning product to it.

CHINA STAINS:

Dissolve 1/4 to 1/2 cupful Diamond Brite™ in a gallon of hot water. Soak the china before washing and drying. If stains are severe, soak the china overnight.

CLEANING BOOSTER:

Adding 1 capful Sol-U-Mel™ to each wash load of baby diapers will remove any offensive odors. Odors are caused by bacteria and Sol-U-Mel™ eliminates bacteria while leaving clothes smelling fresh and clean.

COFFEE STAINS:

Drinking coffee certainly is a Minnesota morning ritual that continues as long as you are home, even if that means right into the evening. If the coffee pot is not on, it is almost on. There is always room for an extra cup or an extra coffee drinker at the kitchen table. I have found that coffee is the ideal drink while playing cribbage. Coffee and cribbage and 15-2's just seem to go together as friends gather to complain about the Minnesota winter. Even in July, the Minnesota-polite-conversation seems riddled with talk of winter and the hopeful, but never materialized reality of not staying around to face another one. "I'll tell you, by golly, I'm not putting up with this snow-stuff anymore..." But, I digress, which is another thing that all coffee drinkers seem to have in common.

After company leaves, you may have coffee cup rings on your kitchen counter or table. Instead of using a lot of elbow grease trying to clean the stains, apply some undiluted Tub 'N Tile™ on the stains. Then rinse with a clean sponge before wiping dry. If you are working with a Formica or fiberglass counter top, rinse immediately. Do not allow Tub 'N Tile™ to dry on the surface before rinsing and wiping dry.

Someday if you're in the neighborhood and want some conversation, a cup of what I think is the best coffee anywhere, and a little pegging mixed in with some complaining about snow and cold weather, well just let me know. I usually have some extra cups and more chairs are always close by, as is an extra can of coffee - if we talk and peg that long.

COMPUTERS & OFFICE EQUIPMENT:

Always unplug anything electrical prior to cleaning. I use ClearPower™ on my computer screens, spraying a little on a cloth to wipe off the built-up dust. The keyboards respond well to cleaning when using 1 teaspoonful Tough 'N Tender™ and 1 capful Sol-U-Mel™ combined in a 32 ounce spray bottle filled with water. It works best if you allow the spray to remain on for a minute or so before wiping off. Typewriters, adding machines and computer keyboards are good "catch-all-sources" for attracting hand and finger dirt. Using this spray leaves surfaces non-magnetic which repels dust.

COPPER:

Have you seen what Tub 'N Tile™ does to tarnished copper? Try the penny test. Dip a copper penny in 1 capful Tub 'N Tile™. If Tub 'N Tile™ will clean a dirty, tarnished old penny, just think what it can do for your copper pots and frying pans. Spray on copper and wipe the grit and black tarnish away.

COUNTER TOPS:

I use 1 teaspoonful Tough 'N Tender™ combined in a 16-ounce spray bottle filled with water to spray my counter top surfaces. All I need do is wait several moments before wiping with a damp cloth or clean sponge. If you have been "allowed to" clean fish on the kitchen counter, or if you have cleaned fish on another counter (even one in the garage), clean the counter with Anti-Bacterial Liquid Soap™. Apply a small amount on a sponge and wipe counter before rinsing off. This will effectively eliminate the fishy smell from your kitchen or garage, provided, of course, you remember to dump the garbage, too.

CRAYON:

Cleaning crayon marks really depends on where the crayon has been marking. For walls, use Sol-U-Mel™ undiluted. Gently try a smidgen of it on the crayon mark, keeping in mind that it can also remove what's under the crayon - such as paint. For clothing, it's another job for Pre-Spot™, particularly if the crayoned-clothing has gone through the washer and dryer before being discovered. It is still possible to remove, but the task is more difficult. Spray Pre-Spot™ on the crayon wax and allow it to stand for several minutes before rubbing fabric against fabric. You may need a small scrub brush or a sharp finger nail to complete the task. If the spot still remains, repeat the process.

CUTTING BOARDS:

Add 1 part Tough 'N Tender™ and 1 part Sol-U-Mel™ to 5 parts water and combine in a spray bottle. Spray this mixture on the soiled cutting boards and allow it to remain for a few moments before rinsing and wiping dry. For additional cleaning recipes for cutting boards, read the preceding recommendations for cleaning counter tops.

DENTURE CLEANER:

Since switching his home to Melaleuca products, Bob soaks his dentures (while showering/shaving) in 1 teaspoonful Diamond Brite™ dissolved in a cup of warm water . After rinsing well, he brushes with Melaleuca's Tooth Polish™. Others recommend other Melaleuca cleaning products, but frankly, I'd proceed slowly especially if your dentures are made with new materials; you could dissolve not only the stains, but also your teeth! Remember, you won't go wrong using Melaleuca's Tooth Polish™!

DESKS:

For dusting, combine a scant half-teaspoonful Tough 'N Tender™ and a dribble or two of Sol-U-Mel™ in a 16 ounce spray bottle filled with water. Spray on a damp cloth and dust. If the desk top has ink stains, apply full strength Tub 'N Tile™ or Sol-U-Mel™ to the ink spot. Repeat if necessary.

DIAPER PAIL:

Use a pail with a lid for soiled diapers. Cover diapers with water and combine 2 capfuls Sol-U-Mel™, 3 tablespoonfuls MelaPower™ and 1 tablespoonful Diamond Brite™. Soak overnight. Wash with 1/8th cupful MelaPower™ and 1 to 2 capfuls Sol-U-Mel™. For whiter diapers, add 1 tablespoonful Diamond Brite™.

DIRT:

I seem to encounter ordinary dirt problems more often than I care to mention. I blame it on excessive gardening and weeding - down on my knees pulling plants and transplanting flowers and bushes. For dirt impacted stains,

I use MelaPower™ full strength applied directly to the dirt stains before adding the garment to my regular wash load. Wash as usual using MelaPower™ and Sol-U-Mel™.

DISINFECTANT SPRAY:

This is a replacement for the heavily-advertised, store-bought disinfectant sprays. Combine 1 part Sol-U-Mel™ with 5 parts water in a spray bottle. It is safer and more cost effective.

If you have any doubts about using this product, as opposed to the sweet-smelling commercial sprays found in grocery store rows, please refer back a few pages to the section on home safety. Some sprays coat your nasal passages with a film that is designed to block your nose from smelling and, therefore, your perception from realizing that something is stinking. While it might be okay initially, have you considered the long-term impact these chemicals may have on your home, family, loved ones, pets - your own - and everyone's health? While this section isn't necessarily a repeat of earlier chapters, I think it's important to realize what the potential impact is of all you do around your home. It is my hope you'll seriously consider the long-term implications of your actions.

DISHES & DISHWASHERS:

MelaDrops™ works far better than any other dish cleaning product I've tried. It's amazing how it works to cut through grease to dissolve food particles. It will not adversely affect your hands and is kind to sensitive skin while being unkind to dirty dishes, pots and pans.

For dishwashers, use 1 teaspoonful Diamond Brite™ if you have soft water and 1 tablespoonful if your water is hard. If you have just converted your home and kitchen to Melaleuca's cleaning products, first run an empty cycle through your dishwasher using 2 to 4 ounces MelaMagic™ and 1 tablespoonful Diamond Brite™. This should help clean out any residue or build-up of old soap and debris.

DOORS & DOORKNOBS:

If you spend most of your time at home like I do, or if you have company as often as I do, your doors and doorknobs probably see more action than - *well, my editors won't allow me to use that analogy here.* But they will allow me to say that since doors and doorknobs are constantly touched, they are also constantly exposed to a wide variety of germs and bacteria. Doorknobs probably pick up more bacteria than almost anything else in the home. I use a 16 ounce spray bottle filled with water, and add 1 teaspoonful Tough 'N Tender™ and 1 capful Sol-U-Mel™. Spray on and wipe dry. Often I use a damp cloth when wiping doors after first lightly spraying them. To remove fingerprints, use a small amount of undiluted Anti-Bacterial Liquid Soap™ on a damp cloth. Rinse with a clean sponge before drying the surface.

DRIVEWAYS:

Many with paved or concrete driveways - who don't live out in the country like I do (where I have a gravel and crushed rock driveway) want their driveways to be stain or spot-free. For them, Brett's "solution" may work. He combines 1 part MelaMagic™ with 8 parts water and 1 to 2 capfuls Sol-U-Mel™, spraying this on any fresh grease stains and then hosing off the driveway with water.

My friend Roswell and I play cribbage at his kitchen table most Tuesday and Friday afternoons. Since he lives on a busy street, I can't park there; his driveway is the only reasonable option. Sometimes after leaving his place, I'll drive around the block just to check, and sure enough, he's out there wiping away any unseen traces of my visit. My old truck's comfortable and fits me well and doesn't, as far as I know, leak anything. I've told Roswell that, but it doesn't seem to stop him. I've even suggested we play cribbage at a neutral site, or at my place, but he keeps insisting I come to his house. Then again, since he's the only one I know who actually sweeps the dirt paths in his vegetable garden, maybe the problem might just be "his" and have little to do with me or my old truck...

DUSTING:

You might think that everyone should know this - but I'm somewhat new to *liking* (really) much of the more mundane housework chores. Now that I've become a Melaleuca customer, I'm discovering things that probably most of you who do housework already know. But, one trick I've discovered is to dust before vacuuming so that any larger debris shaken loose can be picked up by the vacuum cleaner.

Frequently changing the air filter on my furnace also reduces the amount of dust and bacteria particles floating throughout our home. *(Some readers may notice that I referred to the furnace as "mine"; I've learned to do this since the various mechanical apparatus seem to belong to me. This home, however, is always referred to as "ours".)* I like the fact that after I've sprayed and dusted with Tough 'N Tender™ and Sol-U-Mel™, the cleaned surfaces stay non-magnetic and will repel dust and dirt. *For most of my years prior to discovering Melaleuca's cleaning products, I loathed cleaning and dusting and nearly everything domestic. Now, I actually look forward to "dusting" days.*

ELSIE'S TRAVELING TOWELS:

This is a home-made cleaning aid named after the person who suggested the idea to us; we don't know if she developed it, or if it was a mutual decision based on a whole lot of trial and error by many people. Elsie suggests combining 2 capfuls each of Sol-U-Guard™, Sol-U-Mel™ and Clear-Power™ in 16 ounces water. This should create sufficient liquid to fully saturate about one-half of a large roll of paper towels that have been separated and torn apart. Elsie's Traveling Towels are just about the best home-made-all-purpose-cleaner we've ever seen - or used. In warmer weather, I always keep a sealed container in my car's trunk, or in the pickup's tool box, when traveling. Pete tells me they always take along a bucket of Elsie's Traveling Towels in their motor home, and carry a full line of Melaleuca supplies (health and cleaning), too. According to Pete, carrying his fax, computer, enrollment supplies and a showcase of Melaleuca products helps them spend their retirement years making money. Plus, they're happier, safer - and far healthier, too.

FINE WASHABLES:

I do not own anything I would consider a "fine washable". But, Annie claims her recipe is best for washing her finer things. Add 1 teaspoonful Tough 'N Tender™ to a basin of cold water. Gently wash and rinse. Her suggestion is easy and cost effective. After knowing her for years, I know I can trust her judgment on this.

FLOORS:

For linoleum and ceramic floors. Use 1/2 cupful MelaMagic™ in a gallon of water. If using a spray, mix 1 part MelaMagic™ to 8 parts water. Nancy suggests using 6 ounces of Sol-U-Guard™ in a gallon of water to clean stains she terms "moderate" from linoleum and ceramic floor surfaces. I have lived long enough to realize that Nancy's moderate may differ from what I would term "moderate", but by this time, you probably have the idea and will start using less product (you can always add more) in any cleaning remedy and/or suggestion mentioned.

For hardwood floors. Joan has a house full of hardwood floors and a handful of work caring for her young son. She advocates saving time and money using 1 tablespoonful Tough 'N Tender™ in a gallon of water to clean her floors. Sometimes, when company is coming and the floors are not as clean as she would like, Joan combines 1 teaspoonful Tough 'N Tender™ and 16 ounces water. She sprays this on and wipes it off. Best of all, her floors are cleaned quickly and easily.

For hard-to-remove heel marks. Dab Anti-Bacterial Liquid Soap™ on a cloth and rub briskly - but not so brisk as to remove the finish if it's a wood floor. Some recommend using Sol-U-Mel™ on wood floors. However, check a small area first to see how it works, since it could remove the floor's finish, if the finish is not well-sealed.

Maybe you can be as independent as Grandma Johnson who issues her guests paper slippers at the door - asking visitors to go if they're unwilling to leave their shoes (and heel marks) outside. Wearing paper slippers is about the only way to get at a piece of Grandma's state-fair blue-ribbon-award-winning home-baked pie and probably the best coffee in all of Southeastern Minnesota. Folks who know, tell me that Grandma serves a lot of pie...

FLY CONTROL:

Combine 1 teaspoonful Tough 'N Tender™ with 1 capful Natural Spa & Bath Oil™ in a 16 ounce spray bottle filled with water. In areas prone to flies, spray daily for one week, then try spraying 2 to 3 times weekly. To eliminate flies from a porch, deck or yard, be sure to respray after each rainstorm. If you are in an area where deer flies can readily find you, liberally apply Sun-Shades 9™ or 15™.

FRUIT WASH:

These days with all the chemicals poured on fruits, smart consumers (particularly those who have switched their homes to safe Melaleuca products) are rinsing and washing both home-grown and non-home-grown fruits. It takes so little time to wash and rinse our fresh fruits that I think it's probably best to soak almost all of them before eating. In my home, I use 1 teaspoonful Tough 'N Tender™ in a sinkful of water and soak fruit for at least several minutes. I then use a strainer to rinse the fruit off before eating or adding to recipes. *Refer back a few pages to the "How Safe Is Your Food?" section; it mentions that Federal law permits the residues of 67 pesticides to be on strawberries. Strawberries? This sure makes one want to think seriously about buying their berries in a grocery store. . .*

FURNITURE:

For outdoor furniture, use a spray of 1 teaspoonful Tough 'N Tender™ and 1 capful Sol-U-Mel™ combined in a 16 ounce bottle of water. Spray the furniture and scrub as needed. Rinse with a hose or well-dampened sponge and allow to dry in the natural open air.

GARAGE FLOOR:

This suggestion assumes that the garage floor has already been sealed. Brett uses 1 part MelaMagic™ with 8 parts water and 1 to 2 capfuls Sol-U-Mel™. He sprays this solution on fresh grease stains in his garage and concrete driveway and then hoses them down with water. If ever there was an award for clean driveways, Brett would win. His garage floor and driveway are the cleanest in town.

GARBAGE CANS:

Cleaning garbage cans is at the top of my list of least-favored chores. Melaleuca's products make even this task a little easier. I mix 1/2 cup MelaMagic™ and 1 to 2 capfuls Sol-U-Mel™ in a gallon bucket filled with water. Using a long handled scrub brush, I can easily wash both the inside and outside before rinsing. To prevent odor buildup, clean garbage cans every other week.

*I also recycle now. Cans and bottles are rinsed out and separated. Papers go in one bag and food wrappers are kept to a minimum and bagged separately. In milder months, I compost all my food particles and table scraps, believing it is better to add them to my own garden's soil. Developing a routine to separate the garbage my household creates is easy and takes only a few moments each day. When you think about it, if everyone who is physically able would recycle just their own stuff - what kind of world would we have **then?***

GARDEN STAINED HANDS:

Before gardening, apply Body Satin™ Lotion to your hands. This will create a protective coating for your hands and help protect them from stains. When you have had enough gardening for one day, wash your hands with Anti-Bacterial Liquid Soap™.

GLASS:

Use ClearPower™ as directed on the label. I use old newspapers to wipe the glass after spraying. Dennis prefers using terry cloth towels or old cloths of any other sort . See "Windows" for additional comments.

GRAPE JUICE STAINS:

Spray Tub 'N Tile™ full strength. Allow it to stand several minutes. Add 1 tablespoonful Diamond Brite™ and 2 tablespoonfuls MelaPower™ to a gallon of water. Soak the stained item thoroughly before washing it as usual with MelaPower™.

GRASS STAINS:

For almost any types of stain on clothing, use Pre-Spot™ or MelaPower™ as a stain remover. Apply to the stain and allow it to remain on for several minutes before rubbing briskly. Wash as usual. I have also had success using MelaPower™ full strength on tough stains. Apply, rub briskly and soak before washing. If MelaPower™ dries, reapply and wait less time before rinsing.

GREASE (AUTOMOBILE/INDUSTRIAL):

MelaMagic™ is the best product I've found to clean my car and truck engines, the driveway and any grease spots. If you are cleaning a large area and using a bucket, dilute 1/2 cupful MelaMagic™ and fill with water. For cleaning chores around the garage or workshop, I keep a quart spray bottle containing 4 ounces MelaMagic™ mixed with water. **Absolutely always** add 1 or 2 capfuls Sol-U-Mel™ to any chore that involves removing grease!

GREASE (SPOTS/STAINS - PERSONAL):

Have you ever been dining out and looked down and noticed part of your dinner on your tie or shirt? It used to be that friends and family would know where I had been by the variety of food I carried home. Not anymore! I discovered Hot Shot™ Mouth & Throat Spray. It's the best instant spot and stain remover. I spray any fresh spot with Hot Shot™ and rub with a fingernail before rinsing with cold water. *Now my friends have to follow me to figure out where I am catching my "extra" snacks. They can no longer read my clothes.*

GREASE (SPOTS - RUGS/CARPETING):

Anti-Bacterial Liquid Soap™ is an effective spot remover. Use a scant amount and rub on, then rinse off. I've found it works best if you blot rather than rub the stain. *No one will ever know you dropped your lasagna on the hall carpet on your way to the den. Your carpet stain can disappear just as easily as your leftovers.*

GUM:

See Chewing Gum.

GUMMY & STICKY SURFACES:

If your house is like mine, sometimes surfaces become gummy or sticky for no apparent reason. When I find these, I clean them with Sol-U-Mel™ applied full strength. It cuts through the residue gum and effectively cleans all sticky surfaces. This is one area where Sol-U-Mel™ comes to the rescue. *After a day-long cleaning campaign, try to resist running around your house shouting "Hi-Ho-Sol-U-Mel" in praise of Melaleuca's cleaning products. If you live on a street like mine, you will only succeed in waking the neighbors, who by this time are probably not at all surprised at anything they might hear coming from your house...*

HAIR - STATIC ELECTRICITY:

If you've ever encountered problems with static hair - you know, when the strands seem to stick out wherever they choose after you've brushed - here's an easy solution. Why not spray some diluted MelaSoft™ on your hair brush or comb? People who use this claim it works wonders in eliminating the problem. *For myself, I've such few short strands left that I would actually welcome some static hair - or almost any hair - that could stick up and out from my increasingly visible scalp. . .*

HAIR SPRAY - MISDIRECTED:

Did you ever wonder where misdirected hair spray really goes? It may drift over and land on your walls and floor. If there are spots and you cannot figure out the origin, hair spray may be the culprit. To remove, apply MelaMagic™ to a damp cloth and wipe the spots. After waiting a few moments, use a sponge and rinse before drying. If any residue remains, repeat the process. *This is probably the second of two critical areas in your bathroom where "aim" is really important.*

HARD WATER SPOTS:

Use Tub 'N Tile™ full strength for heavy duty cleaning. Spray it on and allow it to remain without drying. Rinse and wipe dry. Do not use Tub 'N Tile on marble surfaces.

HUMIDIFIER"

Use 1 to 2 tablespoonfuls Sol-U-Mel™ in a humidifier's water chamber. It will clean the humidifier while delivering healthy, fresh air throughout the room or house.

INK:

If removing from fabric, be sure to test the color fastness prior to applying undiluted Sol-U-Mel™. To remove ink, use either Tub 'N Tile™ or Sol-U-Mel™ directly on the spot. *If the fabric has been in the dryer before being noticed,* use undiluted Sol-U-Mel™. Some suggest using a different formula that calls for combining 2 ounces MelaMagic™ and 1 capful Sol-U-Mel™ with 8 ounces water. Dab on and rub briskly. The ink should easily lift free of the surface. *HOWEVER:* Make sure the surface having the ink has been sealed. If you are working with untreated wood, the ink stain will likely penetrate and be very difficult to remove. If the stain is on marble, do NOT use Tub 'N Tile™.

INSECT REPELLENT- ON PERSONS:

Our friend Russ, who probably enjoys camping more than any other living person, uses this recipe to repel insects: Combine 1/2 bottle Body Satin™ Lotion with 4 ounces Natural Spa & Bath Oil™ and 4 ounces Sol-U-Mel™. Apply to skin twice per hour. This will keep bugs and ticks off when hiking or staying close to home. Be sure to apply this mixture around your feet and legs since it is an excellent preventative for deer ticks and flies. One of the things Russ likes about this repellent is that it smells good and does not contain harmful petroleum or chemicals. According to him, the proof is in the putting (on). Russ also reports that he sometimes actually smells so good that folks even look forward to him stopping by for an extra cup of coffee and some neighborly campground conversation.

Others recommend using a concoction of 2 capfuls Sol-U-Mel™ combined with 10-15 drops T36-C7™ in a 16-ounce spray bottle filled with water. They claim this is effective in spraying anything outdoors, including the outdoors.

INSECT REPELLENT - PLANTS:

Use 1/2 teaspoonful Tough 'N Tender™ in a 16 ounce spray bottle filled with water. Spray on any plants that have pests.

JEWELRY:

Friends who are "jewelry experts and collectors" report that they dip most of their jewelry (avoid dipping soft stones and pearls) into undiluted Tub 'N Tile™. They rinse the jewelry well before allowing it to dry. Applying several drops Tough 'N Tender™ to a toothbrush also works well. Gently scrub and rinse. Most ordinary jewelry worn throughout the day can be kept clean by immersing hands in the various cleaning solutions suggested in these pages. *As an ardent observer of human behavior, I have learned that anyone who wears tarnished jewelry probably is not doing too much of the cleaning around their home. Maybe some priority adjustments regarding the division of household tasks is needed. Then again, maybe that is better left to another book.*

KITCHEN:

For general daily cleaning chores, add 1 teaspoonful Tough 'N Tender™ and 1 capful Sol-U-Mel™ to a 16 ounce spray bottle filled with water. This is an effective all-purpose cleaner perfect for almost any kitchen surface and situation.

KITCHEN FLOORS:

See Floors.

KITCHEN SINK:

To clean scuff marks out of enamel sinks, use undiluted Tub 'N Tile™. The results are spectacular! Diamond Brite™ is also effective. Wet the surface to be cleaned and sprinkle Diamond Brite™ on the stains. Scrub and rinse. Repeat as necessary.

LAUNDRY:

I use 1 pumpful (about 1/8th cupful) MelaPower™ in an average wash load. If I had a water softener, I would be able to use less MelaPower™ per load. Brett measures the amount of his MelaPower™ in tablespoonfuls. His house has soft water.

LAUNDRY STAINS:

Use Pre-Spot™. It takes out most stains, yet is really gentle on fabrics. To use, spray the Pre-Spot™ undiluted on the stain. Wait a few minutes to allow the liquid to penetrate the cloth, then use a fingernail or firm brush on the fabric. Try rubbing fabric against fabric. Then rinse with çold water and launder as usual. If the stain is still visible, repeat the process a time or two. Almost every stain can be removed by following this recipe.

If I have temporarily run out of Pre-Spot™, I will use undiluted Tough 'N Tender™ on the fabric stain. After applying with a damp cloth, I allow it to remain for a few minutes before rinsing off.

LAWN MOWERS:

Combine 1 part MelaMagic™ with 8 parts water. Spray the mower then wait a few minutes before rinsing. If any dirt or grime remain, repeat the process and use a firm brush to scrub the mower clean.

LEATHER CLEANER:

Sally probably wears more leather (and looks better in it) than any woman I know. She wears her leathers when touring the Minnesota and South Dakota landscape on her Harley. Sally uses 1 part Anti-Bacterial Liquid Soap™ combined with 2 parts water and applies it to her outfit. Scuff marks and dirt easily come off and the leather is undamaged by the cleaning. Sally says this works far better than any commercial leather cleaner she has tried.

LEATHER SOFTENER:

Denny, our attorney, had a favorite old leather vest his bride of 30+ years rediscovered packed away in a seldom-visited closet. The leather was stiff and old and seemingly ruined. But, he told me that since Body Satin™ Lotion worked so well on his feet and hands, he thought it worth a try. Well, within several days of randomly applying the lotion, between his briefs (that's as in legal briefs), the vest became soft and pliable. Denny claims his vest has now made its way into the front hall closet. I've seen him wearing it and I've got to admit, it's just about as soft as Denny's fee schedule. So, if you've an old leather anything, why not try this Melaleuca leather softener, too.

LIGHT FIXTURES:

ALWAYS unplug and disconnect any light fixtures **BEFORE** attempting to clean!

For regular cleaning: In a 16-ounce spray bottle of water, add 1 teaspoonful Tough 'N Tender™ and 1 capful Sol-U-Mel™. Spray on, sponge and wipe dry.

For heavy duty cleaning: Add 1 ounce MelaMagic™ and 1 capful Sol-U-Mel™ to 7 to 8 ounces water. Spray on, rinse well and wipe dry.

For disinfecting: Add 1 ounce Sol-U-Guard™ and 1 capful Sol-U-Mel™ to a 16 ounce spray bottle filled with water. After spraying, leave on for several minutes before rinsing and wiping dry.

LIGHT SWITCH PLATES:

I don't know how many times the light switches in my home are turned on and off each day, but it must be at least several hundred. Some of us are so intent on saving money, that the lights are switched off more I think, than they're switched on. I don't understand how that's done either. You know, switch plates probably gather as many, if not more, germs than doorknobs.

To clean light switch plates, I combine 2 ounces MelaMagic™ with 2 capfuls Sol-U-Mel™ in a 16 ounce spray bottle filled with water. I spray on and let it stand for a few moments before using a damp sponge to wipe the plate clean. This really works on all the switch plates throughout our home, in the garage, shop, outdoors and down in the boat house, too.

LIPSTICK:

Well, if lipstick's on your collar, it may tell some tale on you - or it may be purely incidental. However to remove lipstick, apply Pre-Spot™ according to directions and rub fabric against fabric to rub out the stain. Add 1 to 2 capfuls Sol-U-Mel™ to your regular wash, and launder as usual. You may have to repeat this process several times if the lipstick stain proves difficult to remove.

MARBLE SURFACES:

DO NOT USE TUB 'N TILE™ ON GENUINE MARBLE SURFACES. Instead, add 1/2 teaspoonful Tough 'N Tender™ to a 16 ounce spray bottle of water, spray on and wipe dry.

MAGIC MARKER (ON TILE OR WOOD):

Use undiluted Sol-U-Mel™ for permanent marker stains. Rinse with a wet cloth and dry. Depending on the degree of stain, a second application may be needed. Use Sol-U-Mel™ lightly and then only on sealed surfaces.

Undiluted Sol-U-Mel™ may remove a surface's finish, so be careful when using. Kerrin tells me she has had great success in removing marker stains left by her visiting grandkids. She makes a paste of 1 tablespoonful Diamond Brite™ dissolved in a half cup of hot water and dabs it on with a cloth or sponge, applying it to whatever has been marked. Kerrin mentions that if this doesn't entirely clean the markings the first time, it probably will when reapplied carefully again.

I haven't any first hand knowledge of needing this type of cleaning, but I trust Kerrin enough to know that if she suggests this solution works, it does. So does not having any magic markers in the house when little company and family stop over. You know, there's so many things these days you have to protect little kids from, that some of the more common items found around most homes often escape our notice - until something like a stain or mark has already happened. I've lived enough years to realize that with all that can go wrong, some well-placed marker stains aren't that big a calamity .

I guess this is another example of being thankful for the times when I don't stumble and fall. It becomes an opportunity to appreciate all of the gifts I'm blessed with each day. As I grow older, I find it increasingly important to honor each sunrise and to acknowledge that each new day holds the prospect of new adventures and new moments to excel at whatever it is I am planning to do. It is in the early morning hours of most days, before that first cup of coffee is fully consumed, that I vow to take no prisoners, to play no serious mind games and to make no unreasonable ransom demands on my family and friends. Writing this paragraph reminds me of what my mother would often say in her later years, "I've decided I'm going to take one day at a time. Even if I'm not too sure which day it is."

MIRRORS:

You will *know* who is the fairest of them all if you regularly use ClearPower™ to clean your mirrors. Otherwise, add 2 to 3 drops Tough 'N Tender™, in a 16 ounce spray bottle filled with water. Just spray on and wipe dry. Mirror cleaning was never any easier, or more affordable than this! This is one area of home cleaning that will be reflective of your ability.

MOSQUITO SPRAY:

This is a recipe for an excellent mosquito spray that will not harm your family. Combine 1 teaspoonful Tough 'N Tender™, with 1 capful Sol-U-Mel™, and 1 capful Natural Spa & Bath Oil™ in a 16 ounce spray bottle filled with water. You can safely spray your clothing and outdoor areas. To keep the mosquito population under control, spray often, particularly after rainfall and prior to any evening or dusk-time activities. For other spray recipes, jump back a few pages and read Insect Repellent.

MOTORCYCLES:

Since Sally and Charlie ordered their new Harley, they kept their old bike looking showroom clean by using this method: Combine 2 tablespoonfuls MelaMagic™ and 1 capful Sol-U-Mel™ in a 16 ounce spray bottle filled with water. Spray this on, sponge, rinse and wipe dry. I have heard reports that even an old Norton was made to look showroom clean when its owner used this recipe.

MOLD & MILDEW:

See Bathrooms.

MUD:

When mud is on washable clothing, use Pre-Spot™. If the stains are built-in, scrape off as much of the dried mud as possible. Use either undiluted Tough 'N Tender™ or 1 to 2 capfuls Sol-U-Mel™ on a brush and scrub the mud. Then launder with MelaPower™ as usual.

NON-MAGNETIC SURFACES:

Tough 'N Tender™ applied undiluted to a damp cloth can be wiped on television and computer screens. It repels dust and keeps screens amazingly clean and static free.

ODORS:

For laundry odors: Add 1 to 2 capfuls Sol-U-Mel™ to each wash load. Friends with babies in their homes claim this works particularly well for eliminating the odor from diapers.

For onion odors: Wash hands, cutting boards and counter tops with a small amount of Anti-Bacterial Liquid Soap™.

For pet odors: Spray pet areas and carpet with 1 part Sol-U-Mel™ diluted in 5 parts water.

For smoke odors: In an 8 ounce spray bottle, add 1 to 2 ounces Sol-U-Mel™ and fill with water. Spraying the air will eliminate smoke odors and leave the room smelling fresh and clean.

OVENS:

Use Tough 'N Tender™ to clean ovens. Apply full strength using a cloth or sponge and let stand for a few minutes before wiping dry. Some cooks suggest using 1 part Sol-U-Mel™ and 5 parts water. Use a scouring pad and rinse well. To boost cleaning efficiency, add 1 capful Sol-U-Mel™.

If it has been some time since you have cleaned your oven, you may be "faced" with tough spots that defy normal cleaning. Combine Diamond

Brite™ and MelaMagic™ into a paste and apply it to the spots. Allow it to soak in before rinsing and wiping dry. This paste should handle almost any oven cleaning chore, but if some residue remains, repeat the process.

PAINT - ACRYLIC:

If you have "gone and gotten" it on clothing, spray Pre-Spot™ directly on the paint. Then wait several minutes to allow it to dissolve the paint. Try rubbing the paint with your fingernail or use a firm scrub brush or tooth brush. Rinse with cold water. If any paint still remains, repeat the process as needed.

PAINT - OIL AND WATER BASED:

I am not a painter. This fact is known by all who have watched my painting efforts that seem to cover me with more paint than the item needing it. Before Melaleuca came into my life, I just sort of acknowledged that some clothes would forever have paint stains on them. BUT - not anymore!

Even I have been able to remove paint from clothes after applying Pre-Spot™ to the stain. Generally, after spraying the Pre-Spot on the paint stain, I wait a few minutes to allow it to soak in before rubbing cloth against cloth. After rinsing the garment, if any paint remains, I repeat the process before washing with MelaPower™ and Diamond Brite™.

PANELING:

Clean old-looking paneling by wiping with a cloth dampened with Tough 'N Tender™. Wipe on and dry with a clean cloth.

PIANO KEYS:

If Mozart were still alive, I just know he would suggest you use Tough 'N Tender™ on piano keys. Or, he would tell you that sonata's aside, you should practice by just wiping the keys with a soft cloth dampened with a little Tough 'N Tender™. Then calmly wipe them dry. *And keep practicing, practicing, practicing so that some day your playing will be remembered and taken just as seriously as you now take your cleaning, cleaning, cleaning performance.*

QUICK CLEAN & SHINE:

Use ClearPower™ according to directions. Spray on and buff dry. This works perfectly on surfaces such as mirrors, counter tops and sinks. Others suggest using 1 teaspoonful Tough 'N Tender™ in a 16 ounce spray bottle filled with water. Spray on and sponge to dry.

RUST:

For rust stains on clothes, apply undiluted Tub 'N Tile™. Rub on and allow it to soak before adding the item to the washer. Some suggest that soaking the item in a washer load having 1/8 to 1/4 cupful MelaPower™ is more effective. Another method is to periodically spray a dilution of Tub 'N Tile™ and water on the spots throughout the day. Continue until the rust spots fade, then launder as usual.

SCREENS:

Add 1 tablespoonful Tough 'N Tender™ to a gallon of water; use it to carefully scrub the screen. I have found that it works best to first lay the screen on an old blanket or tarp and work on it there. Use a brush for difficult areas. As you rinse with a garden hose, stand the screen vertically to turn it freely on both sides. Tap and air dry before placing it back on the window.

SCUFF MARKS:

Apply several drops of Anti-Bacterial Liquid Soap™ on a damp wash cloth and rub firmly against the scuff marks. If any marks remain, apply undiluted Sol-U-Mel™ on a damp cloth and use to wipe the marks. Rinse before wiping dry. Repeat as necessary. Caution: Sol-U-Mel™ can remove the floor finish or paint. Try a small area first and then proceed cautiously.

SHOWER STALLS:

Use 1 capful Sol-U-Mel™ as a cleaning booster with 1 ounce Tub 'N Tile™. Combine with 6 to 7 ounces water. Spray the stall area and allow the spray to remain on the stall walls for several moments. Rinse well and wipe with a damp cloth or sponge. If this solution dries before rinsing, repeat the process. Do not use Tub 'N Tile™ on marble.

SINKS:

Use 1 capful Sol-U-Mel™ as a cleaning booster with 1 ounce Tub 'N Tile™. Combine with 6 to 7 ounces water. Spray the sinks and allow the spray to remain on for several moments. Rinse well and wipe with damp cloth or sponge. If this solution dries before rinsing, repeat the process. Do not use Tub 'N Tile™ on marble.

SILVER CLEANER:

Form a paste using equal parts Melaleuca's Tooth Polish and Tub 'N Tile™. This can be applied to silver with either a dry or slightly damp cloth. Let stand for several minutes, then remove using a clean dry cloth. Some suggest substituting Diamond Brite™ for Melaleuca's Tooth Polish. However, I have found that either combination is an effective and safe silver cleaner.

SNOWMOBILES:

There was a time when I traversed the Maine woods, sometimes driving into the Allagash as far as where the logging roads ended and Nugent's Camp, carved out of the woods, lay ten miles across the frozen water. These were the days of snowmobile adventures with business partners Bruce and Charlie and some others from a New England snowmobile association. There were other times when I traveled alone in the more populated areas of Central Minnesota. In these areas, I often rode "lost" (unlike New England where I was never lost). All of those times stretch backwards several decades in a bank of memory that tends to focus only on what was good. Now perhaps because of changing priorities, I no longer ride.

If you snowmobile now, you need to know how to keep your sled looking showroom clean. From all I know about Melaleuca products and snowmobiling, I will suggest that you use this combination. Add 1 capful Sol-U-Mel™ and 1 ounce MelaMagic™ with 7 ounces water. Spray on, sponge to rinse and wipe dry. I am confident that your machine will look as fresh as a late October snow in a quiet woods.

SOFTENER:

Now that we've converted our home to Melaleuca products, I can rest assured that we no longer are challenging the universe environmentally. An added bonus is that our home is safer, and we are saving money on our cleaning supply purchases, too. An example of this savings comes from using MelaSoft™ at laundry time. I add 1 or 2 tablespoonfuls to the final rinse on an average load. If I forget to add it during the final wash cycle, I can always add 3 to 4 squirts in the dryer drum. If you are reluctant to do that, spray some MelaSoft™ on a wash cloth and toss that in the dryer along with your clothes.

SPILLS:

It was our turn last year to host the family's Thanksgiving dinner and the 23 invited became the 31 who attended. There is always room at our table for extra chairs and Lord knows we have enough dishes and silverware to take care of nearly any number of unanticipated arrivals. Everything was going well until one of us (who just happened to be carrying the gravy boat from the kitchen to the dining room) slipped or tripped. All eyes watched the gravy leap into the air before splashing down on the carpeting. There was more gravy in the kitchen, so no guest went without gravely because of the mishap, but the cleanup became a family-style event since several Melaleuca-product-experts were in attendance.

This is what they did to solve the gravy-stain-into-the-carpeting problem. Some white terry cloth towels were supplied and one was dipped into a mixture of 1 teaspoonful Tough 'N Tender™ combined with water in a 16 ounce spray bottle. This was sprayed on the stain and blotted, beginning at the outside edges and working in a clockwise motion towards the center. Another dry cloth was used to wipe up the spill, again working in a clockwise motion beginning at the outside. After this, all the moisture and wetness were blotted up and the area was rinsed again. Another clean white terry cloth towel covered the area, so that whenever something was needed from the kitchen, it required one large step to pass over the spot.

After giving thanks, and after consuming bellies full of good food shared with great company, family and friends and several new acquaintances, and some good conversation, the towel was removed. Not a single sign of the earlier gravy that splashed into the carpeting remained. I would have to say that this dinner was probably one of the best we ever hosted. I do not necessarily recommend this type of crisis, but it did serve a greater purpose in bringing everyone together in a common cause. When you think about it, even clean carpeting is something to be thankful for, as is a table-full of friends and family sharing conversation and selves. Maybe this is in part what Thanksgiving is all about. . .

STATIC CLING:

Always look in the mirror before leaving home. After you arrive is probably too late to realize that whatever it is you are wearing is tucked up higher in the back than your prevailing modesty should allow. If you wear a garment that sometimes is "grabbed" by static cling, lightly spray MelaSoft™ directly to the underside of the dress or skirt. This will alleviate the problem and allow the material to fall naturally.

TAPE ON WINDOWS:

I am not sure why some people put tape on their windows, but I know that Sol-U-Mel™ will remove it. Wipe undiluted Sol-U-Mel™ across the tape and pull it off. Most all tape's adhesive will break-up and come off with Sol-U-Mel™. Bob suggests full strength Tough 'N Tender™ as the better product choice for this chore.

TAR (ON CAR):

After our last trip back from Maine, the family car returned with considerable tar buildup on the grill and front end. I believe this was due to the many miles of road construction we drove through in Ohio and Pennsylvania. I tried Sol-U-Mel™ full strength on the grill and used a mixture combining 1 part Sol-U-Mel™ with 5 parts water for the car's fenders and hood. When that still left some spots, I used Sol-U-Mel™ full strength. The tar came off quickly and the paint was undamaged. I then hosed off the car and proceeded to wash it as usual.

TAR (ON HANDS):

T36-C7™ applied full strength takes tar off hands. Wash afterwards using

Anti-Bacterial Liquid Soap™ and dry.

TELEPHONES:

Next to doorknobs and light switches, telephones are generally overlooked when it comes to cleaning. Routinely now, I include my telephones on my weekly cleaning ritual. I use a spray of 1 ounce MelaMagic™ combined with 1 capful Sol-U-Mel™ and 7 ounces of water. I spray on and sponge rinse before drying.

TOILET:

Spray Tub 'N Tile™ full strength, let stand for several minutes before scrubbing clean. Professional toilet scrubbers first turn off the water valve, flush and empty the toilet tank and bowl, and then apply undiluted Tub 'N Tile™ to the built-up stains. Diamond Brite™ sprinkled on a sponge or scrubbing pad is also effective. To rinse, turn the water back on and flush several times. If any stains remain, repeat the process. (Refer back to the "Bathroom" listing for additional tips.)

TOYS:

As much as adults are susceptible to transmitting bacteria and germs from handles and doorknobs to ourselves, this is minimal when compared to what can be transmitted child-to-child from exchanging and handling each other's toys.

Toys are often in the mouth, sometimes in the yard, and always on the floor. Each of these are places where germs and bacteria thrive. Toys that respond to washing should be soaked in a sink or tub of water to which 1 capful Sol-U-Mel™ and 1 teaspoonful Tough 'N Tender™ have been added. After the toys soak, rinse well before toweling dry. They will then be ready for more play, more experiences shared, and much more washing and cleaning.

TUBS:

In an 8 ounce spray bottle, add 2 ounces Tub 'N Tile™ and 6 ounces water. Spray on and allow to stand for several minutes before rinsing off. If this mixture dries before rinsing, reapply and wait less time before rinsing off. Remember, Tub 'N Tile™ is a "no-no" on marble surfaces.

UPHOLSTERY:

Always check the manufacturer's cleaning instructions prior to cleaning any upholstery or upholstered furniture. If they're okay and you've decided you're going to do the cleaning chores yourself, try adding up to 1/2 capful

Sol-U-Mel™ and 1 capful Tough 'N Tender™ in a 16 ounce spray bottle filled with water.

This makes an ideal all-purpose upholstery cleaner. Then slightly dampen a cloth and apply it to the upholstered item. Sometimes a firm nylon brush also works particularly well when cleaning arm rests. This procedure should remove most of the surface dirt without causing harm or stress to the fabric. However, be careful that you don't get the backing or filling wet. After cleaning, rub the upholstery with a clean, dry cloth. For stains, spray again and gently wipe the upholstery clean.

If you have soft water, decrease the amounts of Melaleuca products added to the spray bottle. Some suggest you cut quantities by at least 50%. Rinse carefully and rinse well, as any cleaner remaining on the upholstery will only attract more dirt and buildup of grime.

Always test the color-fastness of any upholstery before you start cleaning. Try applying a small amount of cleaning solution to a very small area before attempting to clean the whole piece.

Vegetable Wash:

These days, with all the chemicals used in raising vegetables, it's important for everyone (particularly for those who have switched their homes to safe Melaleuca products) to rinse and wash home-grown and store-bought vegetables. It takes so little time to wash and rinse the foods, that I believe washing all produce is a really important way to safeguard my family and myself from unnecessary exposure. As a vegetable wash, I use 1 teaspoonful Tough 'N Tender™ in a sinkful of warm water and keep all vegetables in it for at least several minutes. I then use a regular kitchen strainer and rinse the foods off before using or refrigerating.

Writing this makes me realize, once again, that I am assuming the water from our kitchen faucet is safe water. Thinking about water quality leads me to believe there's probably a whole other book waiting for someone to write. If there was a practical book that told how to improve the quality of our own water supply, and how America could have an unlimited abundance of good drinking water supplies to last forever, I'd buy that book, too. . .

Vinyl:

Follow cleaning suggestions under "Leather Cleaner".

Walls:

For heavy-duty cleaning, dilute 4 ounces MelaMagic™ in a gallon of water.

For general cleaning: Combine 1 teaspoonful Tough 'N Tender™ and 1 capful Sol-U-Mel™ to a 16 ounce spray bottle of water.

For heavy duty cleaning: In a 16 ounce spray bottle, add 1 to 2 capfuls Sol-

U-Mel™ with 1 to 2 ounces MelaMagic™, fill the bottle with water and shake to mix or blend.

For disinfecting: Combine 1 ounce Sol-U-Guard™ and 1 capful Sol-U-Mel™ in a 16 ounce spray bottle filled with water. For additional information, see "Ceilings & Walls".

WINDOWS:

Use Clear Power™ on glass as directed. When cleaning windows some use old towels to wipe the windows clean and dry. However, these can leave streaks and lint behind. Paper towels will work, but they cost money and then need disposal. This is why I prefer using ordinary newspapers. There is no lint and a fresh supply arrives every morning. Considering costs, it appeals to my frugal nature, too.

WOOD FLOORS:

On the hardwood floors in our dining room and kitchen, I add 1 teaspoonful Tough 'N Tender™ to a half-gallon pail of water and use a long-handled sponge mop. After wetting the mop and squeezing out the excess water, I lightly "skimmer" over the floors. Then using a dry mop, its easy to buff the surfaces. I use this same measurement for preparing a dusting/cleaning solution to use when wiping down the woodwork around the doors, cabinets and windows and on the wider window sills where our cats seem to prefer sleeping. This solution of mostly water really works as it cleans and leaves the surfaces dust free. Best of all, it won't harm the animals - or my family. Please refer to an earlier section on home safety for additional reasons it's important to use Melaleuca products for all home cleaning chores.

ADDENDUM

For additional information on this subject, I'll refer you to another S.T. Clark® book that details home safety and offers more home safety facts. You can order your copy of "S.T. Clark's® How Safe Is Your Home?" from its publisher - Compton Park Companies, Inc., 222 Little Canada Road, Suite 175, Little Canada, Minnesota 55117. Or, call their 24-hour toll-free telephone order line for Visa or Mastercharge - 1-800-826-7932. This book, as all S.T. Clark® books, is also available from Gaughan Fisch, Inc. (publisher of this book); order number appears on inside back cover.

TESTIMONIALS

"*Rather than write a dozen letters with each one telling about another use my group has discovered - and attempting to have you send us a dozen books - we've decided to just send in our one-page list. So here goes.*

"*I have found that if I use a lotion (such as Body Satin™ Lotion, Hand Cream™ or Problem Skin Lotion™) after rubbing on Pain-A-Trate™ or T36-C7™, my skin will stay nice and soft and won't dry out. Penny, who's a nurse, developed an effective bedsores treatment by combining equal parts of Sol-U-Mel™ and Spa & Bath Oil™; she just dampens a cloth and holds it on the sore for several minutes before applying Mela-Gel™ or another lotion. Several of us have experienced bleeding guns and have learned that by rinsing with Breath-Away™ Mouth Wash and then brushing carefully with Tooth Polish™, our gum problems are alleviated; we also repeat the Breath-Away™ mouthwash rinse after brushing. Joan's children are still of an age to get chicken pox; from first hand experience, she now knows that if she rubs undiluted Spa & Bath Oil™ on the pox sores, healing is often accelerated. For congestion relief, Albert advocates the use of Pain-A-Trate™ liberally rubbed on the chest; follow this with a covering lotion. My grandson uses this as an effective treatment for his twin's diaper rash - Tough 'N Tender™ as a bubble bath; just combine scant quantities in warm bath water. And, here's something that S.T. should really recommend for his diabetic readers. My husband has had tremendous results using a foot soak that combines 1 to 2 capfuls Nature's Cleanse™ in a pan of warm water. He hasn't yet got out the ice chest that S.T. talks about using, but I expect that will be next. Anyway, hope you can use some of these and pass them on to your readers. Your book is certainly enjoyable! I'll be ordering another 100 copies next month, too!*"
                                                                        -NRT, California

"*I'm really impressed with Melaleuca's home care products when cleaning my stove's oven. I've found that by simply diluting some Tough 'N Tender™ with water, I can spray the oven's inside surfaces. Then I use a spatula to take-off the hard-to-remove spots and also use warm water and a brush. Sometimes, I also spray Mela-Magic™ on hard-to-break-apart spots. What I really like best of all is that I NEVER have to use a mask or rubber gloves with Melaleuca's products. They're safe to use, VERY cost effective, and they really work!*"
                                                                    -R.G., Washington

Farm Facts

Farmers across America are discovering new uses for Melaleuca alternifolia oil in their day-to-day operations. They are developing treatment options and obtaining results most people would find amazing. Many farmers now routinely use products containing the oil to treat their livestock.

Melaleuca products consistently deliver a lower cost-per-application than nearly any other remedy. Saving dollars means more revenue directed to areas other than costs. Adding operational savings together, can often turn a break-even year into one that's profitable. Today's capital-intensive farming operations necessitate that farmers use products that will save time and money. This is a simple economic lesson that directly relates to the reasons why large numbers of farmers are now converting to Melaleuca products.

As in all other treatment suggestions contained in this book, individual results will vary. Results achieved depend upon factors and conditions, many of which cannot be controlled. These can include temperature, quality of water and accurate measurement of product.

If you use treatments and remedies different from what I have listed, please let me know. I will try to include your suggestion(s) in a future edition. You will receive a complimentary copy of the first edition in which your suggestion appears. If similar suggestions are received, the first one that crosses my threshold and is used, will receive the free book.

General Facts

Ant Killer:

Spray undiluted Pre-Spot™ to all areas where ants tend to "congregate".

Ant Preventative:

Combine 2 ounces Sol-U-Guard™ with 8 ounces water and spray all "ant-prone" areas.

Fly Control:

Combine 1 teaspoonful Tough 'N Tender™ with 1 capful Natural Spa and Bath Oil™ in 16 ounces water. Spray the animal area and animals daily for 7 to 10 days. Then spray weekly until the fly problem is under control. Do NOT spray directly into an animal's face or eyes.

Jon tells me he prefers using 2 capfuls Sol-U-Mel™ and 10 drops T36-C7™ added to a 16 ounce spray bottle filled with water. He claims his best results come from spraying all barn and stall confinement areas at least several times weekly.

For personal use, one can apply Russ' previously mentioned combination. Blend together 1/2 bottle Body Satin™ Lotion, 4 ounces Natural Spa & Bath Oil™ and 4 ounces Sol-U-Mel™. Since this works for Russ when he is camping in the great outdoors, it may also prove beneficial for farmers. Why not try it and see if it will work for you?

Jon's brother Tim uses a different recipe calling for 2 to 3 ounces Sol-U-Mel™ added to a pint of water. He sprays this to eliminate flies in his horse and dairy barns. I would advocate using a weaker mixture to start, testing it for killing ability as I gradually add more Sol-U-Mel™. If a stronger mixture is necessary, more Sol-U-Mel™ can always be added.

Gosh, we're sorry this eradication method probably won't work where the weather is year-'round nice. We call our proven method by several easy-to-remember names: Winter, Ice, Sub-Zero Temperatures, Snow and Wind Chill. You folks in the far southern and western regions of the country do not have the same advantage as we do in this part of the country. We indeed consider ourselves most fortunate and blessed to have such an effective method, one that really works, and one that can virtually eliminate all flying critters - for months at a time.

Mosquitos:

If you cannot wait for the cold air and winter to arrive, liberally apply Sun-Screen 9™ or Sun-Screen 15™ to all body areas that may be exposed. Leonard and Elsie both advocate the use of either product to keep these little flying critters away from them, especially while finishing their daily list of chores. For additional insect-control recipes, read Fly Control.

Farm Equipment

Bulk Milk Tank:

Pour 8 ounces of undiluted Tub 'N Tile™ in the water-filled bulk tank and let soak for 10 minutes. An alternative method some dairy farmers suggest is to spray the tank using undiluted Tub 'N Tile™. The tank's walls will shine and look nearly new when wiped with a towel. However, some areas may require more soaking. Rinse the tank thoroughly with water after cleaning. Run sufficient clean water through the tank until the water clears of any foaming. Repeat this at least several times before filling the tank with milk again.

COMBINE WINDOW CLEANER:

This works well for any enclosed cab implement. Add 1 tablespoonful Tough 'N Tender™ to a gallon of water. Scott told me he carries a 16 ounce spray bottle under the combine's seat. He cleans the windows at least every 2 to 3 hours when in the fields. 5 ounces ClearPower™ combined with water in a 16 ounce spray bottle is also effective. It seems to "discourage" dirt and dust buildup. However, it does cost more per use than the few pennies cost of Tough 'N Tender™.

MILKSTONES:

The first time you clean the milk lines, fill them with undiluted Tub 'N Tile™. Allow this to soak for about 10 minutes before pumping the Tub 'N Tile™ through the system. Repeat five consecutive times. Each time you clean the milk lines thereafter, use 1 part Tub 'N Tile™ to 5 to 10 parts water. Always run sufficient clean water through the lines to rinse them well. All milk lines must be clean and free of any cleaner, before starting to run milk through them again.

MILK TANK CLEANING:

To clean exteriors, use equal parts Sol-U-Mel™, Sol-U-Guard™ and Tough 'N Tender™ combined in water. To clean tank interiors, use a "scant" amount of Sol-U-Mel™ (since it foams) in a few tankfuls of water for line and interior cleaning. Melaleuca products are safe and non-toxic. However, always rinse lines especially well after completing cleaning and before running milk back through again.

PRESSURE WASHING:

Hand clean the area before soaking with the proper mixture (according to directions) of MelaMagic™. Let this solution soak for 2 to 3 hours. Then finish the cleaning using the same mixture.

For newer washers that have a small hose, use undiluted MelaMagic™ (try about 1/2 gallon every 2 hours).

In older washers with a tank hookup, combine 1 quart MelaMagic™ with 24 gallons water. To boost cleaning, add 3-4 tablespoonfuls Sol-U-Mel™ to the cleaning solution you are using. Be sure to run adequate amounts of clean water through the lines before re-using.

UNDER THE HOOD CLEANING:

The standard suggestion I have heard most is to use MelaMagic™ according to directions. My friend Rodney tells me he sprays undiluted Pre-Spot™ under the hoods of his farm equipment. He claims this makes it easy to wipe the grease and grime away.

CATTLE

CATTLE - CASTRATION:

For best results in healing the cut site, follow the remedies and recipes listed just below under Cattle - Cuts, Scrapes, Burns.

CATTLE - CUTS, SCRAPES, BURNS:

Use the Spray Mixture (In a 1 gallon bucket, combine 16 ounces Sol-U-Mel™ and 4 ounces Tough 'N Tender™; then fill with water to spray injured area twice daily until the areas affected have healed. Fence burns and any cuts and scrapes can be serious if left untreated or under-treated. If a more severely injured animal will allow you in close enough to treat it, apply one of Melaleuca's ointments or creams. T36-C7™ is always effective when used on injuries. Cement burns on the knees are common to cattle. If knee swelling occurs, apply liberal amounts of T36-C7™ and follow with Pain-A-Trate™. Continue treating until the injured area has healed.

CATTLE - DEHORNED INFECTIONS:

Combine 4 tablespoonfuls Tough 'N Tender™ with 2 capfuls Sol-U-Mel™ in a gallon of water. Flush the infected area using a syringe. After flushing, sprinkle T36-C7™ on the infected area. Repeat daily as necessary.

CATTLE - HOOF ROT:

After cleaning, wrap the hoof with a clean strip of towel or cloth. Either before or after wrapping, soak the covering thoroughly using 1/2 to 1 cup Tough 'N Tender™ and 2 to 3 ounces Sol-U-Mel™ diluted in water. Try to keep the strip in place for at least 7 to 10 days and re-soak it as often as it seems necessary. For severe cases, use 16 ounces Sol-U-Mel™ and 4 ounces Tough 'N Tender™ to a gallon of water.

CALVES & COWS

CALF BIRTHS - DIFFICULT:

As soon as the calf is born, place 5 to 10 drops T36-C7™ down each nostril, and 5 to 10 drops on the back of the tongue.

CALF COUGHING:

Spray undiluted Sol-U-Guard™ into their bedding at least once weekly. Spray more often if you think it is necessary.

CALF - GENERAL PNEUMONIA:

Apply 10 drops T36-C7™ in each nostril and 6 drops on the back of the tongue. Continue for 7 to 10 days as necessary.

CALF - ON MILK REPLACER:

To assure that calves are receiving their necessary vitamins and minerals, dissolve 3 Vita-Bears™ Children's Vitamins in a cupful of milk and add it to their warm milk replacer.

CALF - PENS - MANGE:

Wash out the pen using a garden sprayer. Then spray down the bedding using 1 ounce Sol-U-Guard™ mixed in 16 ounces water. By spraying the bedding once a week, you should be able to keep the mange under control.

CALF - PNEUMONIA IN NEWBORNS:

Place 10 drops T36-C7™ in each nostril once daily until the calf recovers. Also rub some Nature's Cleanse™ around their nose and mouth.

CALF - SCOURS:

Twice daily (morning and evening) orally administer (using a syringe) 1 ounce Nature's Cleanse™ diluted in 4 ounces water. Continue treatment until the calf's bowel movement firms up. ***Do not give Nature's Cleanse™ undiluted!***

CALF - UNTHRIFTY:

Dissolve 3 Vita-Bears™ Children's Vitamins in milk and add to the calf's milk both in the morning and at night.

COW - HIP & JOINT INJURY:

Tom reports that one of his cows injured her hip on the barn while heading outside for some sunshine. The wound became severely infected and the top part of her hip bone was destroyed. Nothing used to treat her seemed to work until he cleaned the wound and applied 1 undiluted capful of Nature's Cleanse™. He then followed with applications of T36-C7™ and Triple Antibiotic Ointment™. Tom reports that the infection cleared and the wound healed within several days following these treatments.

Tom also reports that his vet was at the farm doing routine herd checks and stated that seldom has he seen such a severe injury heal. More frequently, he told him, the injury becomes infected resulting in the destruction of the joint. When this happens, the producing cow is reduced to hamburger and freezer meat. *Which also comes in handy to feed a growing family, but as Tom says, you hate to give up on a good milk producer. . .*

COW - INFECTION FOLLOWING BIRTH:

For infection following birth due to retained afterbirth, Jeremy reports success using 1 to 2 ounces Nature's Cleanse™ diluted in a quart of water. According to him, this will help kill any infection that's present. He claims this formula can be adjusted for the particular weight and condition of any animal and will work for most every farm animal having a similar condition.

COW - MASTITIS:

Apply liquid Pain-A-Trate™ liberally to the infected quarter twice daily. Continue treatment until the cow is free of infection. If mastitis is severe, first apply liberal amounts of T36-C7™. Follow with liquid Pain-A-Trate™. For outbreaks of herd mastitis, mix 1 ounce Sol-U-Mel™ with 10 ounces water, mix well and use as a teat dip.

COW- MILKING TIME:

This is Jon's favorite recipe that he developed and it is now used by several large dairy farmers in Illinois, Wisconsin, Iowa and Minnesota. For a milking time teat wash: Combine 1 quart Tough 'N Tender™ with 1/2 quart Sol-U-Guard™ in a gallon container, then fill with water. Be sure to mix together to blend well. Add 1/2 ounce of this mixture to a gallon of wash water. Jon tells me this recipe is an effective and safe teat wash for use at milking time.

SPRAY MIXTURE - ALL PURPOSE:

In a 1 gallon bucket, combine 16 ounces Sol-U-Mel™ and 4 ounces Tough 'N Tender™. Then fill bucket with water and use as a spray.

SPRAY MIXTURE - ON CHAFED OR SORE TEATS:

Spray 2 to 3 times daily until they have healed. An alternative suggestion is to apply 2 to 3 drops T36-C7™ daily until healing sets in. Refer to the suggestions under Cows - Milking Time.

SPRAY MIXTURE ON UDDER EDEMA OR FRESH UDDER:

Spray udder twice daily. Pain-A-Trate™ has also been very effective in treating fresh udder.

Spray Mixture on Udder Sores:

If sores appear between the quarters, or between the udder and the leg, spray a liberal amount on the area. Repeat at least twice daily until the sores have fully healed.

Teat Cuts:

Triple Antibiotic Ointment™ applied to teat cuts and sore teats will most often provide quick healing. Many dairy farmers are discovering just how effective Melaleuca oil, and products containing the oil, are in their routine cow and calf care. Others are "experimenting" using various strengths and combinations of Sol-U-Mel™ and Nature's Cleanse™.

Teat Spray:

Spray a mixture of 1 ounce Sol-U-Mel™ combined with 5 ounces water. Respray after washing. Be sure you have sprayed the teat ends, too. Refer to other suggestions in this section.

Udder Wash:

This recipe comes from the heart of Southwestern Wisconsin's prime dairy country. Combine 1 quart Tough 'N Tender™ with 3 quarts water. Use 2 ounces of this mixture with 1 capful Sol-U-Mel™ added in 5 to 10 gallons water. Prior to putting on the milkers, spray the udders with a mixture of 1 part Sol-U-Mel™ combined with 5 parts water.

CHICKENS

Chickens - Coccidinosis:

When chickens are away from their bedding, spray it using 1 ounce Sol-U-Guard™ in a quart of water.

Chickens - Egg Room Salmonella & Aspergillus

Spray weekly using 1/2 ounce Sol-U-Guard™ in a quart of water.

Chicken House - Fogging Barns:

Use *up to* 1 ounce Sol-U-Mel™ to every 5 ounces water.

Chicken House - Salmonella:

Salmonella grows in the general house area and in the chickens where it can spread to their eggs. To kill salmonella, use either 1 ounce Sol-U-Mel™ or Sol-U-Guard™ in a quart of water to spray their house. This should kill **most bacteria including salmonella. CAUTION: Always avoid all direct contact between the birds and the spray.**

CHICKS:

To reduce the incidence of respiratory disease, place 3 to 4 drops Sol-U-Mel™ into the small drinking water reservoirs. Use 2 to 3 tablespoonfuls Sol-U-Mel™ in a 500 gallon reservoir.

CHICKS - SICK CHICKS:

If you think the chicks need an extra boost, my friend Charlie Poore suggests adding a scant single drop of Sol-U-Mel™ in 32 ounces water. He suggests limiting this treatment to once in any 2-week period.

DOGS

DOG - HOT SPOTS:

So-called "hot spots" and body abrasions respond well to applications of T36-C7™ when applied frequently. Using this reduces their pain and prevents infection while promoting healing. Use Mela-Gel™ if drying or scaling results.

DOG - MANGE:

Apply T36-C7™ to the bare or scant hair areas where the dog has scratched the hair off. Use ProCare™ Professional Pet Shampoo regularly to help prevent mange. Another preventative is to make sure your dog is on Melaleuca's ProCare™ Nutritional Treats for Dogs.

DOG - ODOR:

This is for those who really care how their pooch looks and smells. If your dog sleeps with you, or sleeps at the foot of the stairs, or guards the house from the kitchen floor (over there by the door), you probably care how your dog smells. *You could treat your dog to a shampoo using any of Melaleuca's human-shampoos, but Gold-Person and my household like her better when she is treated to a session with ProCare™ products. I know you will feel better and sleep better when your dog smells - well, more un-dog-like.*

DOG - PAW ABRASIONS:

Paw abrasions can be treated with Mela-Gel™ or Problem Skin Lotion™. Dogs do not like the smell or the taste of Melaleuca oil, so they are unlikely to lick it off. Repeat applications several times daily as necessary.

Dog Versus Skunk - Skunk Winning:

When Rover comes home with an accompanying odor that smells mainly of a tangle with the wrong end of a skunk, one thing is certain, he cannot come back indoors and sleep on the kitchen floor as usual. The next thing that is certain is that you have an unusually demanding cleaning chore that needs some immediate attention. My South Dakota friends tell me that what has worked best for them - and for their Rover - is to run a large outdoor tub full of water and bring out the Anti-Bacterial Liquid Soap™. *It absolutely will deodorize the pooch - and whatever the pooch has been in contact with - including you.* Repeat if necessary. However, this should work with only one application. *Really.*

Hogs & Pigs

Hogs - Coccidinosis:

When out of the pen, spray bedding with 1 ounce Sol-U-Guard™ combined with enough water to fill a quart spray bottle.

Hog Confinement - Cleaning:

Combine 32 ounces MelaMagic™ into 24 gallons water. Use this in your pressure washer to clean walls and ceilings. This spray should eliminate mold re-growth after just one treatment. Another suggestion is to make a spray using 1 ounce Sol-U-Mel™ in a quart spray bottle filled with water. Use on all walls and ceilings.

Hog Confinement - Salmonella:

When hogs are not in confinement areas, spray using 1 ounce Sol-U-Guard™ combined in a quart of water.

Hogs - Disinfecting Udder at Farrowing Time:

Use 1 ounce Sol-U-Mel™ with 20 ounces water.

Hogs - Fogging Barns:

Use up to 1 ounce Sol-U-Mel™ with 5 ounces water.

Hogs - House:

For disinfecting, use 1 ounce Sol-U-Mel™ to 30 ounces water. Some hog farmers recommend a slightly stronger mixture.

Hogs - Mastitis:

This remedy can also be used when the sows are holding their milk. Apply T36-C7™ to the bag followed by liquid Pain-A-Trate™. I have talked with several farmers who "insist" that liquid Pain-A-Trate™ seems to work better when T36-C7™ is applied first.

Hogs - Pens - Mange:

Wash out the pen using a garden sprayer. Then spray the bedding using 1 ounce Sol-U-Guard™ combined with 30 ounces water. Routinely spraying the bedding every week should keep the mange under control.

Hogs - Salmonella in Barns:

Spray the barn with a solution of 1 ounce Sol-U-Guard™ and 30 ounces water.

Hogs - Sow Wash:

Spray the sow using a mixture of 1 teaspoonful Tough 'N Tender™ and 1 capful Sol-U-Mel™ combined in a 16 ounce spray bottle filled with water. Spray the crates using 1 ounce Sol-U-Guard™ with 30 ounces water.

Little Pig - Greasy Pig Disease:

At least daily rub the pigs down with Body Satin™ Lotion. If this does not alleviate the problem, you may have to apply the lotion 2 to 3 times daily until the condition is cleared.

Little Pig - Itch Problems:

To reduce itch problems, mist the little pigs with a sprayer or sprinkle them with a water can using a mixture of 1 ounce Sol-U-Guard™ with 50 ounces water. WARNING: Treating the animals more than once per week may cause them to develop flaky skin.

Little Pig - Post-Weaning Scours:

Add 1/2 cup Sol-U-Mel™ to a 500 gallon water tank. J. Bruce suggests wiping T36-C7™ or Nature's Cleanse™ liberally on the mother's teats. He says that this helps the little pigs nurse-in the Melaleuca alternifolia oil as they get their milk. Nursing pigs can also be helped by making a paste of dissolved Vita-Bears™ Children's Vitamins and water. Just paint it on the mother's teats before nursing.

Little Pig - Respiratory Problems:

To reduce respiratory problems, mist the farrowing pens daily with 1 ounce Sol-U-Mel™ combined with 5 ounces water.

HORSES

Paul and Doris, our neighbors near the park, probably understand both ends of a horse better than anyone. They've furnished most of the following information. Doris prefers treating their animals with Melaleuca products and claims that nearly every external ailment responds and can largely be alleviated when the oil is used. Paul asked me to tell readers that to use Melaleuca alternifolia oil in routine and preventative horse health care procedures and not to wait until something minor becomes more serious. Consider this as you're being told.

HORSE BREEDING:

Before breeding, wash the mare and stallion with Nature's Cleanse™. Follow accompanying dilution directions. Using Nature's Cleanse™ should help reduce the bacteria count while increasing the opportunity for conception. **Never give any products containing pure Melaleuca oil internally to horses.**

HORSE - BREEDING MARES:

Nature's Cleanse™ helps eliminate the risk and is not a spermicide. Use it diluted according to directions to wipe down a stallion. It cleans, deodorizes and is more mild than any other product available on today's market.

This is not to suggest that Melaleuca advocates the use of Nature's Cleanse™ in the treatment of horses, particularly in their "accompanying literature." You must assume some responsibility for "reading between the lines" to calculate the quantity of concentrate that should be used. Base your decision on factors you know such as the animal's size, health, weight, quality of the mix water, temperature and other conditions your horse may suffer from, or be susceptible to developing. Remember that as you use any Melaleuca product, less is often better.

HORSE - CUTS AND ABRASIONS:

For soreness on the outside corners of the horse's mouth caused when biting up, use T36-C7™ and Mela-Gel™. For other cuts, wash the area with Anti-Bacterial Liquid Soap™ and warm water. Towel dry before using cotton to apply T36-C7™ and Mela-Gel™. Repeat this process daily until the wound heals. As the wound is healing, repeat this procedure every other day for several days.

If the animal is touchy about your attempts at doctoring, try to get in close enough to spray the wound with a solution combining 2 teaspoonfuls

Nature's Cleanse™ and 1/2 teaspoonful T36-C7™ combined in a 16 ounce spray bottle of water.

Another treatment suggests combining in a 16 ounce spray bottle of water, 1-1/2 capfuls Sol-U-Mel™, 1 capful Natural Spa & Bath Oil™, 1 capful Nature's Cleanse™, and 2 drops Anti-Bacterial Liquid Soap™. Mix well and spray several times daily .

HORSE - DRY CRACKED HOOF WALLS & HEELS:

Combine 1 teaspoonful Nature's Cleanse™ and 1 teaspoonful Natural Spa & Bath Oil™ in a 16 ounce spray bottle filled with water. Spray the hoof walls and soles.

HORSE - FLY CONTROL IN STALL AREAS:

Use a 16 ounce spray bottle and add 1 teaspoonful Tough 'N Tender™ and 2 ounces Sol-U-Mel™. Spray liberally, making sure you have first covered and protected the horse's eyes and face from any spray. Never spray directly towards the horse's head.

HORSE - GIRTH ITCH (AND OTHER FUNGICIDAL OR PESTICIDAL SKIN IRRITATIONS):

Mix 2 teaspoonfuls Nature's Cleanse™ in a 16 ounce spray bottle filled with water. Apply spray directly to irritated areas.

HORSE - SORENESS ON MOUTH CORNERS:

Use a cotton swab to apply T36-C7™ to the sore areas. After this starts to dry, apply Problem Skin Lotion™.

HORSE - SPRAY MIXTURE - ALL PURPOSE:

In a 1 gallon bucket, combine 16 ounces Sol-U-Mel™ and 4 ounces Tough 'N Tender™. Fill with water, mix thoroughly and use this as a spray for problem areas.

HORSE - SPRAY MIXTURE - ALTERNATE RECIPE (1):

This alternative-all-around spray mixture should be made-up in advance and kept on hand for treating skin irritations: Combine 2 to 3 drops T36-C7™ with 1 teaspoonful Natural Spa & Bath Oil™ and 1/2 teaspoonful Nature's Cleanse™ in a 16-ounce spray bottle filled with water. Many experts suggest using distilled water because it's mineral-free and the purest form of water possible.

Horse - Spray Mixture - Alternate Recipe (2):

This is an alternative-all-around spray mixture: In a 16-ounce spray bottle, combine 1 to 2 drops T36-C7™ and 2 drops Anti-Bacterial Liquid Soap™ with 1 capful **each** of Natural Spa & Bath Oil™, Sol-U-Mel™, and Nature's Cleanse™. Fill the bottle with distilled water, or water that's been brought to a boil and allowed to cool, and shake well to make sure that everything is well mixed. Then spray as directed or needed.

Cuts, Scrapes, Burns:

Use the Spray Mixture on the injured area twice daily until healed. Fence burns and any cuts and scrapes can be serious if left untreated. If an injury is more severe than mild, try to apply one of Melaleuca's ointments or cremes. T36-C7™ is effective when used on almost any injury.

Root Rot:

Use the Spray Mixture. If the feet are severely affected, clean and trim the hoof(s). Spray twice daily until healed.

Ringworm:

Use the Spray Mixture to spray the infected area daily until healed.

Horse - Sunburned or Chafed Udders:

Use Sun-Shades 9™ lotion; those who know tell us they haven't found anything better on the market. Plus, the young colts don't seem to mind the flavor. This works well to treat sunburned noses, too.

Horse - Tack Area Cleaning:

Melaleuca's laundry and cleaning products work best in cleaning tack areas. They are mild, safe and can be used to sanitize and deodorize almost any area. Many people advocate using Anti-Bacterial Liquid Soap™ as a leather cleaner. Some suggest a 50-50 mixture, others claim that dabbing the soap on the leather and wiping off with a damp sponge works best.

Horse - Thrush:

For minor thrush, combine 2 teaspoonfuls Nature's Cleanse™ with 16 ounces water. In more severe cases, mix 3 teaspoonfuls Nature's Cleanse™ with 16 ounces of water.

TURKEYS

TURKEY HOUSE:

Mist the empty turkey house weekly. Use 1 ounce Sol-U-Mel™ combined with 5 ounces water.

TURKEY HOUSE - SALMONELLA:

Salmonella can grow and spread in the turkeys and spread to their eggs. To kill salmonella, use 1 ounce of either Sol-U-Mel™ or Sol-U-Guard™ combined with 30 ounces water. Spraying the room should kill most bacteria including salmonella. Always avoid any direct contact between the birds and the spray.

TURKEY LINE FLUSHING:

When the water system is not in use, flush all water lines using a mixture of 2 capfuls Sol-U-Mel™ combined with 1 tablespoonful Tough 'N Tender™ and 5 gallons of water. Let the lines soak overnight and then flush well with plain water. Sol-U-Mel™ tends to create a good quantity of foam, so repeated flushings may be necessary.

NOTE:

Missing from this listing are conditions and treatments for elk and white tail deer, llamas, sheep, mink, fish, goats, ostriches and a few more "farm animal" categories. As of this writing, I had not received any reliable information from any farmer on the care and treatment of these creatures. Future editions may well include other comprehensive farm animal care information.

FOOD FACTS

There are dangers in the home that concern the foods we eat. According to Bill Moyers in a March 30, 1993 Frontline report, "In the past five years alone, farmers have dumped over five billion pounds of insecticides onto their crops, more than 11 billion pounds of herbicides into the soil, almost two billion pounds of fungicides - all in an escalating war to ensure good harvests. And, like in any war, civilians caught in the middle are the first casualties."

In this same report, Mr. Moyers also stated that, "A recent National Cancer Institute study found that if you live on a farm, you have a far greater chance of getting some forms of cancer." And, "There are concerns that pesticide residues (in our foods) are disrupting such basic biological processes as the endocrine, nervous and immune systems." And, "Federal law permits the residues of 67 pesticides in strawberries. The EPA suspects that seven may cause cancer." And, "The farmer is not the only one responsible. We consumers are part of the problem, demanding the cosmetically perfect fruits and vegetables that chemicals produce. Did you know that many of the chemicals used have nothing to do with protecting crops? They merely make fruit bigger, shinier, more pleasing to the eye."

Rachel Carlson, author of *Silent Spring*, and one of the first to raise questions about the long-term effects of agricultural poisons on humans, said in the same Frontline report, "We have to remember that children born today are exposed to these new chemicals from birth, perhaps even before birth. Now, what is going to happen to them in adult life, as a result of that exposure? We simply don't know."

So what can each of us do? It might help if we do not insist on buying perfectly formed produce with bright, appealing colors. Organically grown fruit usually is not perfectly shaped. Sometimes the color is darker than the color we have become accustomed to finding in well-fertilized fruit. The appearance of the outside is not as important as the fact that organically grown fruit has never been chemically treated. Eating an organically grown apple for example, allows one to taste the apple instead of tasting the chemical residue left over from aggressive growing techniques. Even if the chemicals and fertilizer cannot be readily tasted, they are still lurking somewhere in the fruit.

We can also wash all our store-bought (and farmer's market or roadside purchased) produce in 1 teaspoonful Tough 'N Tender™ and a pan-full or sink-full of water for several minutes before eating.

ADDENDUM IN CONCLUSION

In this book, I have attempted to blend the facts of Melaleuca alternifolia oil with an injection or two of humor and perhaps a few remembered tales from some of my life's experiences. My favored editorial tone is one that has been described as "conversational". Through these pages, I have asked for your comments and other product use suggestions; I am serious in seeking your responses.

If you are not a Melaleuca customer and would like to try these products, contact another customer in your area. If someone has given you this book to read, talk to them. Melaleuca people can be found almost anywhere. And I know, one will be absolutely delighted to talk with you!

To my way of thinking, it's really not too important how you come into Melaleuca. What is important is that you convert your home and life to safer products that are better for you and cost less money.

The first printing of this book was originally released November 15, 1993; by the time of the next printing, there was so much additional information that the book was rewritten and expanded to its current 144 pages. Since then, each printing has had some revisions and corrections. This edition offers major additions and changes, also. Over the past several years Melaleuca has had one of their most popular cleaning products both discontinued and reintroduced; we've tried to keep pace, finding recipes that could work as replacements, sort-of, and advocating their use. The company's reintroduction of Sol-U-Guard® presented both another challenge and an opportunity. By removing the replacement recipes, we found some space to talk about the miracle of super-antioxidants. This, then, is the 3rd major revision of the book and the 15th printing.

I particularly want to take a few lines here to thank all of you who have contributed ideas and alternative product-use suggestions, treatments and chore solutions. So, thank you! Many readers' comments have already been incorporated in this book, others are waiting for more space to showcase their stories and product-use suggestions. Still, I encourage you to send in your letters and ideas; they are important to presenting the "great facts" about this remarkable oil, and to telling the Melaleuca story. And remember, if your idea or suggestion is the first like it received, and if it's included in a future edition, you'll receive a complimentary copy of the first edition in which it's printed.

Many use this fact-filled book as their working reference and resource guide; they write in it, circle what they like and add other data as it's learned. So, why not do the same? Simply keep your own copy of "S.T. Clark's® Great Melaleuca Fact Book" close by, where you can find it when and as you need it.

Well, together we have arrived at this book's ending lines. As I close my words, I assure you that all is still well here. I hope things are the same at your place, too.

S.T. Clark®, November, 1996

BIBLIOGRAPHY

Blackwell, A.L., *"Tea Tree Oil and Anaerobic Bacterial Vaginosis"*, 1991, The Lancet

Brouse, R.O., *"Melaleuca: Nature's Antiseptic"*, 1992, Sunnyside Health Center

"Controlling Type II Diabetes", 1983, Krames Communications

DeGroot, A.C., Weyland, J.W., *"Systemic Contact Dermatitis From Tea Tree Oil"*, Dept. of Dermatology, Carolus Hospital; Dept. of Cosmetics, Regional Inspectorate for Health Protection; "Contact Dermatitis", 1992

"Diabetes A to Z", 1988, 1992, American Diabetes Association

"Heather's Household Hints", 1993

Humphrey, M.A., *"New Australian Germicide"*, 1930

Igram, C., *"Killed On Contact"*, 1992, Literary Visions Publishing

Kalowitz, G.L., *"The Effect of Essential Oil Type on the Setting Time of Grossma's Sealer and Roth Root Canal Cement"*, 1991

Lappe, M., *"Germs That Won't Die"*, 1992, Anchor Press/Doubleday; and "Chemical Deception", 1990, Sierra Club Books

"Melaleuca Alternifolia", 1985, Essential Oils Data Search, Inc.

Olsen, C.B., *"Australian Tea Tree Oil"*, Kali Press

Pena, E., *"Melaleuca Alternifolia Oil: Its uses for trichonomal vaginitis and other vaginal infections"*, 1962, Obstet Gyunecol

Penfold, A.R., *"Melaleuca Alternifolia (Cheel)"*, 1925, Royal Society of New South Wales Journal; and Penfold, A.R., & Morrison, F.R., *"Tea Tree Oils"*, 1977, Robert E. Kreiger Publishing Co.

Sokol, N.G., *"Poisoning Our Children"*, 1991, The Noble Press

"S.T. Clark's® Diabetes & Melaleuca Alternifolia Oil", 1995; *"S.T. Clark's® Health To Wealth"*, 1995; and *"S.T. Clark's™ How Safe Is Your Home?"*, 1995, Comptom Park Companies, Inc. (Order Line: 1-800-826-7932)

Standards Association of Australia, *Australian Standards for Oil of Melaleuca Alternifolia*, 1985.

Swords, G., & Hunter, G.L.K., *"Composition of Australian Tea Tree Oil"*, 1978, Journal of Agricultural Food Chemistry

"The Wonder From Down Under", and the Melaleuca Starter Kit, Melaleuca, Inc.

Tong, M.M., Altman, P.M., Barnetson, R.StC., *"Tea Tree Oil in the Treatment of Tinea Pedis,"* 1992, Australas J. Dermatrol

Walker, M., "Clinical Investigation of Australian Melaleuca Alternifolia Oil for a Variety of Common Foot Problems", 1972,   Current Podiatry

INDEX

TESTIMONIALS

"I have been doctoring for nearly three years with a variety of prescribed medication, trying to get rid of a fungal infection under my toe nail. After only four weeks of daily applications of T40-C5™, I saw positive healing results. Now after just four months of daily applications, my toe nail again appears completely normal."

M.W., Minnesota

As a veterinarian, I am using Melaleuca products, including T36-C7™, to heal wounds and ulcerations on animals in my care. The results are worth mentioning; I intend to write a longer letter, and perhaps submit some of my research on this. Melaleuca has made a difference in the lives of my patients. Maybe that's the best compliment any product can have, that it makes a difference in someone's life. I hope by using Melaleuca, I too, will make a difference."

-B.C., Wisconsin

"Just a quick note to tell you how much we enjoy your book! Since you asked for suggestions and comments, here's one I use: My pets are tropical fish and I've had problems with the green growth or build-up in their tank. So I got to thinking about which Melaleuca product might be the best one to use in a very-diluted form. I think I found something that may work for other fish owners: I used a drop of Nature's Cleanse™ in my tank's system. It doesn't appear to adversely affect the fish, yet it quickly cleans away all of that slime-like green buildup that seemed to appear in the tank system."

-B.W., New York

TESTIMONIAL ADDENDUM

Testimonials printed throughout this book represent a fraction of the letters we've received. None were solicited; all came from those who just wanted to share something they had discovered with others they will never meet, who may have an interest in hearing their stories.

If you've had success using a particular Melaleuca oil product, why not let us know? Just send us your written comments on a card or letter; your words will be considered for a future edition. (We reserve the right to edit or excerpt.) And if your letter is printed, you'll receive a complimentary copy of the first edition in which it appears. So why not write and tell us how Melaleuca oil has improved your life?